John Hartig

The Final Exit
Medical Assistance in Dying
MAiD In Canada

Second Edition 2024
Collated, Edited and Written
By John Hartig
Cover Design by John Hartig

Published on Amazon and Kindle
with thanks for the chance
to publish affordably,
and for the helpful phone chats

Table of Contents

Dedication

This book is dedicated to the people I knew before, who sadly passed away. Two who used the service of MAiD, medical assistance in dying. Matt Scholtz and Adam. And two who might have used MAiD if it had been available at the time. My former-brother-in-law, Ken Janzen, and my dear sister, Renate Hartig.

I'm not sure if MAiD is a good thing in all circumstances as the qualifications for its use broadens. I can quite understand how this is a merciful and needed medical practice in Canadian society. I traced its evolution, becoming legal in 2016 in Canada. Hopefully, this book is educational, informative, and also touches my readers' emotions about what the people I once knew went through who suffered and died.

Whichever way our medical profession saves lives and also ends them, *Time* is the great leveler of us all. Coming to terms with that fact and accepting it is something we all must also come to terms with throughout our lives.

But at my back, I always hear,
Time's winged chariot hurrying near.
Andrew Marvell 1621-1678

1

The Count Down

Matthew G. Scholtz

April 6, 1946 - June 19, 2023

Three more days to live. I do not know if Canada's recent option for the elderly and the sick to exit this world is merciful or cost-effective to save the government money. Maybe, it's both. I can see MAiD, i.e., Medical Assistance in Dying, gaining more traction in Canada as time goes by. After all, we are changing its mandate and the parameters which are included.

I suppose it is a merciful choice since it is monitored by professionals and painless, like going to sleep. Our government does not have the funds to care for its increasing elderly population. It costs a lot to prolong lives. That's a hard reality. There are some cases where the situation is obviously terminal and the pain so chronic and intense that the sick person is grateful for a way out, that Canada offers a choice like Medical Assistance in Dying.

I started my writing on Friday evening, June 16, with scattered thoughts, the day after I got the e-mail from Matt on Thursday, that he decided to die, rather than live with the miserable after-effects of his cancer treatment. Three more days then to Monday, June 19th, at 11 a.m. when Matt would say goodbye to this world!

Matt will be on the third floor of his apartment with the windows open so he can hear the bagpipes play from the pergola below at his Oxford Estates residence in Tillsonburg. Another tenant John Skinner, dressed in full Highland dress, volunteered to play the bagpipes in honour of Matt. The weather so far is cooperating. It's going to be a sunny day. It must be so hard on his wife, Leni, and Matt's two sons, Stephen, and Andrew.

*****

It is 10:30 a.m. now, this Monday morning. Since I am a writer, I use my imagination of the scene in that third-floor apartment where Matt is being prepped by a doctor who is methodically setting up his equipment. I imagine a nurse standing by, with Matt's wife, Leni and two sons, Stephen, and Andrew, crying, not wishing to be in the way. What I can't imagine is the emotional turmoil the family is going through. Meanwhile, for other people, life goes on.

My wife, Marjorie, went to the back yard to pull weeds this morning as I began writing this first chapter of my new book, The Final Exit. What was happening in Tillsonburg, I asked myself.

My wife interrupted this query because life here in Vineland has to go on too. She wanted a compost bag brought out to her, so she could stuff in the weeds she'd been pulling. I dutifully held the bag open and then took my e-bike to church. I've gotten into the habit of bouncing my basketball off the church wall, catching the ball after one bounce, then flinging it back off the wall for my next bounce. It's the double bounce which makes this exercise the hardest, so for now, my shoulders had to get used to the regular motion of a simple single bounce.

Motion, any kind of motion is good for an aged body. A police car was parked in the church parking lot. I suppose he was more concerned about speeding cars zooming down Menno Street, than about some old geezer on an e-bike bouncing a basketball off the back of the church. I only lasted 15 minutes. During that time, the sun shone on my shoulders, and it felt good. It felt good to be alive.

When I got back into the house, my wife reminded me to do the leg exercises where I cross my bad leg over the other and bend down to loosen up my hips. I took her advice to do just that after I put my e-bike away. I could see my wife through the back window pulling out the weeds methodically and stuffing them into the compost bag. I am lucky that we have an arrangement where she allows me to write and to spend time on the computer to watch old movies too. I will have to do the dishes though before she comes back into the house to make lunch.

So, people go on with their lives, their own little things from day to day. What is Matt doing now? Only another 10 minutes to go until 11 o'clock. Last gestures of love, final words? How difficult all that must be. I wonder whether what I am writing here is worthwhile. Do I need to say all this? Maybe, it brings out empathy in other people, to identify with another human being's pain.

I first got to know Matt and his brother, John, when I was in grade 8. They lived down the street from me on Courtland Avenue. Matt was already in high school at St. Jerome's in Kitchener. I would be there after the summer ended, my grade 9 year. Matt had organized a baseball team, the Vigilantes, for kids around the neighborhood. We played at Victoria Park with hardballs which we scavenged from the tips that the KW Panthers made, where the high ones flipped over the fence onto the road behind the stadium.

Matt, his brother, and a few others of us would keep a keen eye out for these balls which arced over the fence onto the road during evening games at the park. We'd snag the ball and run like hell before the bat boys came out to retrieve the ball, maybe catch us and beat us up for stealing. Well, we figured a foul ball over the fence was fair game! I suppose Matt and John also must have had an in with the bat boys who let them get away with some of those expensive baseballs. Matt and John were the only ones who wore cleats on their baseball shoes, maybe inheriting them as discards from the bat boys with whom they made friends.

Those Saturday morning or afternoon games at Victoria Park were a treasured memory. Matt, Mike Forte, and Danny Glover were the few who could pound that ball over the distant trees at the end of the field. That was an automatic homer. The bigger boys used "Old Faithful", which was a heavy bat with a chip out of the end, but boy, did it have a heft to it. I remember when we chose the name for the team, "The Vigilantes". We were so proud to be part of the team. I think it was Matt who chose the name. It sounded rebellious and daunting.

Well, it's 11 o'clock...a moment of silence...

*****

I suppose it's over by now, 11:15. I don't know. Did Matt hear the bagpipes through the open window? Did he feel a cool breeze come in through the window as "Amazing Grace" was played?

I imagined Leni and Matt's sons holding his hand as he slipped off into dreamy unconsciousness. Perhaps, that's merciful after all. I could understand his decision not to keep living with the misery of pain and having to be fed through a feeding tube. I was not expecting this turn of events though. Matt was supposed to live for another decade. I think he was still in his 70s. I got Matt's e-mail on Thursday morning, June15, only 4 days ago. Here it is:

> My recovery from January's cancer surgery went well.
> for a time.
> Then it didn't.
>
> What I am left with is no quality of life.
> Deaf in left ear.
> Pain in swollen left check
> Can't breathe through left nostril.
> Need a feed tube for most meal because I can't open my mouth very well.
> Food from feeding tube gives me constant diarrhea.
> and sometimes makes me vomit.
> And poor Leni has to deal with all these life's changes, and has become extremely stressed.
> So, I entered the MAiD program.
> On Monday morning, June 19th at 11 a.m.
> I will make my final exit in Apt. 306-83 Rolph Street
>
> So, Goodbye my friends
> Matt

☐

*****

It's time for me to break away from these heavy thoughts and bounce my basketball off the church wall once more. My wife is still weeding in the back. I will have to do dishes when I get back. So far, she hasn't fired me.

The sun felt good as I bounced the ball off the church. The feeling reminded me of John Denver's song, "Sunshine on my shoulders makes me happy."

My wife is dealing with another problem now that she came back into the house. The dishes are done, so I'm off the hook for that. I can hear my wife's frustration as she deals with the Samsung representative on the phone because we cannot get any volume on our TV even at level 80. We have to turn the TV off for a couple of hours and then the volume comes back on, but for how long? They won't replace the TV. It's only 9 months old.

Well, Matt is beyond such concerns, no more talking to techs, no more weeding, no more aches and pains. It's time to help my wife with lunch.

2

Celebration of Life

I have a friend who is 85 years old. He would check the obituaries on the Vineland Tallman Funeral Home website to see if there was anybody listed there whom he knew. He would attend the funeral and often the luncheon afterwards. I used to tease him, that he'd get a free meal out of it. He laughed. "That's not why I go. It's to show respect and to chat with all the people I used to know." Indeed, he knew many people in the Mennonite community within the Niagara Region He'd been a well-known icon in the community for many years.

My brother-in-law Ken Janzen died at home in a hospital bed after combating lung cancer for 9 long painful months. The family was by his bedside when he breathed his last. It was a sad day in winter, January 18th, 2008. The family physician came by to declare Kenny dead. Shortly afterwards, the Tallman Hearse showed up. The gurney was pulled out and Kenny was put into a body bag. He was carefully carted out the door on the gurney, loaded into the hearse. The next time we saw Kenny was in a coffin at the Funeral Home.

I remember the viewing and the reception afterwards at Tallman's where little sandwiches, cookies and drinks were provided and prepared by the ladies in our church.

I understand that Matt was cremated right after the MAiD procedure. All in one day! Existence and non-existence to order Since he was a believer, I pray that he assumed a heavenly body with no cancer and no pain.

I attended a "celebration of life" for my old high school orchestra conductor recently, a celebration which was held shortly after Mike died. His kids paid for the event held at Bingeman Park in Kitchener, a costly affair. Lots of drinks and sandwiches.

I was asked to do some photography since I'd served that function some years earlier at Mike's 75th birthday party and produced some nice photos. My wife sat at a back table by herself and let me roam to snag a photo here or there. Old man Lawrence Bingeman came over and sat beside my wife. I photographed him and his grand niece sitting together and e-mailed them the photo later.

This celebration of life was like a reunion. It was a good chance to meet people whom I hadn't seen since my old high school orchestra days.

Matt's family, I understand, will have a celebration of life as well at a later date. I'm hoping that we don't have doctors' appointments then, so we will have the opportunity to chat with old friends. I never met Leni, Matt's wife.

While MAiD was dealing with Matt, my own family was busy here in Vineland, going on with our own affairs. I'm usually stooped over my computer desk, either writing or watching black and white movies on YouTube. I also love watching my Sci-Fi shows on TV, the digital channel 49-3.

We don't have cable or satellite, simply free TV through the air waves. A Star Trek Marathon was planned for the whole weekend on a rotation basis, so that if you missed one movie, you could catch it the next time around. The movies depicted an older Captain James Tiberius Kirk who was aptly now promoted to Admiral, but still wanting to get command back of the Enterprise, NCC 1701. Spock actually died in one of the movies but got regenerated through a Genesis project. Hard to believe that Dr. McCoy held Spock's "katra" in his mind. As a writer myself, I can imagine the fun the script writers of these movies must have had.

So, Friday evening, Saturday and Sunday went by, knowing that Matt would leave this world on Monday morning. To the poet, T.S. Elliot, April may have been the cruelest month, but to Matt's family, the cruelest month must have been June, specifically June 19th. I still could not believe that at 11 a.m., Matt said his final goodbye. Later that day, he had already been cremated. How quick was that? Did the flames burn away his cancer and all his pain? Leni and Matt had not been married that long. Matt's first wife, Betty, died of cancer too.

I knew a couple in our church who have really been blessed. Walter and Helen invited the congregation over on Saturday afternoon to celebrate their 70th wedding anniversary. Walter got married when he was 21 years old. He'd been born in Ukraine where all that trouble with Putin is happening now. He was fortunate to come to Canada to start a successful life as a contractor.

My wife's Opa and Oma made it to 65 years of marriage, which also was a good milestone. There have been some people who have retained their health and lived long and happy lives. Doesn't the song say, that's just the way it goes? Marjorie and I will have passed our 37th wedding anniversary on August 5th, the same day as her deceased brother's birthday. Birth and Death. Existence and non-existence. Non-existence now on the menu,"to order"!

On Sunday late afternoon, our family met at Marjorie's dad's house in Fonthill to celebrate his 94th birthday...and incidentally, Father's Day. Waldemar, better known as

Wally, was born in Saskatchewan. His family moved East, to Ontario, specifically the Niagara Peninsula, where he became principal of Green Acres school in Stoney Creek. Oma and Opa, in the meantime, did what they did best. They farmed and knew all about orchard trees. They were Mennonites and knew how to work hard, inbred with a good Mennonite working ethic.

Marjorie's sister, Marilyn and husband, Jerry, drove down from Orillia for this milestone event at dads. They brought their little dog, Paisley, along with them. Paisley entertained Sean and Rachel's kids, who are Ethan in grade 10 and Liam in grade 7. Ethan was talking with his grandpa Jerry about getting a guitar. Liam is less interested in music.

I told Ethan that my hero is Jim Croce who composed a lovely song, "Time in a Bottle," way back in 1973 before he died in a plane crash at the age of 30.

The meal for Father's Day was great: Thai food with a "Too Tall Cake" from M&Ms for dessert, all gluten free. There used to be a time when gluten free foods tasted like cardboard, but manufacturers have improved gluten free foods immensely! The minority of people with food allergies are thankful. One has to wonder though, what is the cause of this growing sensitivity to gluten; how has that come about?

3
Matt's Playlist

I'm glad that Matt's kids launched a blog through Caring Bridge, so that friends and relatives could encourage Matt along his journey through that operation on the tumor in his left sinus area and later his radiation treatment.

Things were going so well at the beginning. When things went wrong and Matt let everyone know about his decision to die, Sean O'Sullivan, a family physician for many years, asked if Matt's friends and relatives might want a playlist of songs appropriate for his funeral. I went gung-ho over the idea and forwarded a whole bunch of suggestions, too many. I liked the idea of "Songs for Matt."

I stayed up late into Monday morning scouring the internet for songs which were soothing and a comfort to Matt's family. I came up with suggestions like: Goin' Home sung by Libera, You Raise Me Up by Josh Groban, and Calling All Angels by Jane Siberry. Frank White who also thought of Calling All Angels confessed that these lines touched him deeply in that Siberry song:

> Oh, but if you could, do you think you would
> Trade it all, all the pain and suffering?
> Oh, but then you would've missed the beauty of
> The light upon this earth and the sweetness of the leaving.

Since I'm a musician, a former violin player in the St. Jerome's High School Orchestra, I couldn't resist making more suggestions than poor Sean, whose idea this originally was, could handle. Still, I thought these suggestions were good, something I'd like to be played at my own funeral. Here's the list and that's only half of it!

O mio bambino caro by Puccini, Amazing Grace by John Newton, By the Sleepy Lagoon by Eric Coates, All We Are is Dust in the Wing sung by Kansas, The Long and Winding Road by the Beatles, Claire de Lune by Debussy, The Young Prince and Princess by Rimsky-Korsakov, Gymnopedie No.1 by Erik Satie, Lark Ascending by Ralph von Williams, played by Hilary Hahn, Time in a Bottle by Jim Croce, Someday Over the Rainbow sung by Judy Garland, The Lord is my Shepherd sung by the Tabernacle Choir and of course, Brahm's Lullaby.

Of late, I've also become enamored by oriental singing. I love the minor arpeggios characteristic of Chinese songs. The song Jasmine Flower sung by Teresa Teng is so lovely it made me cry. Though I understood none of the words, the romantic melody and the emotion in Teresa's lovely voice touched my soul.

This playlist does not mean anything to most people. I mean, lists are boring! You have to know the music and the lyrics to touch your heart.

YouTube makes these songs so accessible to a person. It makes one realize what a talent human beings have for creating poetry and songs all over the world. What a wonderful gift music is to us from our Creator.

I've often said in this time of political strife, if only all guns would be turned into cameras and if only people like Putin would learn to play an instrument.

I must admit that I've often wanted to give God a piece of my mind once I get "there". Why did he ever create mosquitoes or insidious diseases like cancer? But then, if all our prayers were answered, wouldn't God merely become a slave to our wishes? God is not a genie in a bottle, and we are not the masters!

When my brother-in-law Kenny died so young, at the age of 37, the family prayed so hard, so very hard, and nothing happened. He died anyway. It's easy to blame God, even Adam and Eve. The human tendency is to look for someone else to blame. God, we say, should save us from our sorrows. We hope for a God; we may even blame him for not existing if that's the way we feel. And when all is said and done, we have to swallow the hard pills that life gives us, no matter what, even if we did not ask to be born. Yet, we should be grateful if we experience a day of sunshine and another person's love.

My brother-in-law's death was so hard on the family. I tried to write a poem, pleading with God: "If you will not take a prayer/ will you take a tear?" No other words came. No poem. My mind went blank. I felt God was too far away to listen, attending to distant galaxies, too busy planting the seeds of stars, too busy in interstellar space, to pay attention to our family's needs...but I prayed anyway.

The suffering we went through slammed my ability to reason and crumbled my Faith. Faith seemed insufficient. What was the sense in praying to a God who might not be there? How could you prove the logical existence of God, even though Thomas Aquinas tried to do just that with his "Quinque Viae".

I do not want to grapple with the "God of the Gaps" to reason out how science fills in the missing pieces until there is no more room for God or for Faith. What Kenny's death taught me was that there is still the "God of the Needs". You believe simply because you need to believe;

you believe in something beyond yourself, simply because you need to.

A decade ago, I used to attend Tuesday morning prayer meetings at the church. An older lady, Betty, was confident: "I know where I'm going. I'm ready to go." Despite her self-assurance about being ready to die and being ready to go to Heaven, I observed that I wasn't quite so sure. "It's the transition which gives me pause," I said. "I'm afraid that the transition will involve pain, which I do not want to accept." I told her that a sickness or disease is not the way I want to go to the other side. If only everyone could die, falling asleep painlessly! But that is not the case. We all need to step out on our own individual journey in a transition that hurts! Our loved ones will have to accept their own journey someday too. It's not a simple matter of being ready, as Betty insists, when the process of getting to the other side will involve a disease which will kill us!

*****

Matt is gone now, and he no longer needs to deal with the trials of this world, with its silly politics, its wars and sicknesses, and its general messiness.

Goin' home. Goin' home. I'm a-goin' home.
Quiet, like some still day, I'm just goin' home.
It's not far, just close by, through an open door.
Work all done, cares laid by, goin' to roam no more;
Mother's there 'xpecting me, father's waiting, too,
Lots of folks gathered there, all the friends I knew.

4
Life Goes On

It surprises me how parallel our lives were, Matt's and my own life. He was born in Czechoslovakia in April 1946, moved to Germany and then to Canada. I was born in Austria in February 1946 and moved to Canada in 1954 with my family, as refugees, as DPs, displaced persons, what the Canadians called us back then, in a pejorative sense. Matt and I were the same age, 77 in 2023.

I've forgotten how I actually met Matt and his younger brother, John. Kids along Courtland Avenue liked hanging out at Victoria Park. Since Matt and his brother, John, lived just down the street, it wasn't surprising for me to end up playing with them in those Saturday morning baseball games.

As I mentioned, we'd play with the hard balls that we'd steal when the KW Panthers knocked a foul ball over the fence onto the road. We'd snatch and run.

We got away with this most of the time. Occasionally, the bigger bat boy would catch one of us and we'd get roughed up a bit for stealing the ball. Since the KW Panthers were semi-pros, those baseballs must have cost a lot.

Matt and John, I think, befriended some of the bat boys who must have given them discarded old baseball shoes with real cleats which helped you to run and take off to first base like the roadrunner. "Old Faithful", which had a chip chewed out of its end, was Matt's favorite bat. He could knock a ball over the trees at the back of the field. Smacking the ball over the trees meant an automatic home run. Matt was one of the few who had the strength to send that ball into the distant foliage. We'd yell, "automatic!"

Keith Kueneman and I were satisfied with just getting on base. Let the sluggers, like Matt, Danny Glover, or Mike Forte, be the stars. Ah, those were the golden days of our youth!

The week before Matt e-mailed me about ending his life through MAiD, I was watching disaster movies, the end of the world kind of stuff. A well-done one was "Supernova", Part 1 and 2, on YouTube. Peter Fonda was in it as the genius professor who predicted that the sun would expand and engulf our planet. We'd become extinct like the dinosaurs. It's interesting how people act in extreme circumstances, rioting in the streets and even the government creating underground shelters in which only the elite would be chosen and saved.

It's ironic but mankind may yet self-destruct, be the maker of its own extinction and not need a natural phenomenon like a supernova to do the job. My wife is not interested in doomsday. Doomsday, if it comes, would take care of itself. She would say, if I had a terminal sickness, watching end of the world movies would not be my choice of a last pastime.

Somehow, with the state of political affairs in the world, Armageddon has become a distinct possibility. Putin has already mentioned nuclear weapons several times if the West keeps helping the Ukrainians.

Thank God, I'm too old to join any man's army. When I was young enough to join, I was exempt because I lived in Canada, and I even roomed with a U.S. draft dodger at McMaster University.

In the United States, in those days, you'd better be smart enough to be in university so that you didn't have to fight in the Viet Nam war. Even then, I was so naïve. I loved pubbing and was smart enough to keep my grades up. The war in Asia did not concern me. I grew long hair, lived the lifestyle of a hippie for a while and bought a motorcycle. How groovy was that? How naïve!

Now that I am 77 years old, I watch Bachelor Father and Father Knows Best on antenna TV on early morning reruns. Channel 11 has My Three Sons on sometimes. The dads were respectively, a lawyer, an insurance exec, and an engineer. What were these shows feeding the ordinary public? My dad was a forklift driver on construction. I earned my way through university by mixing mortar for bricklayers during the summer. The whole array of family/comedy shows was not feeding the public anything realistic. But some administrative guy thought these themes were perfect for people to watch on TV.

*****

I wish that Matt was still alive so that I could chat with him about immigrants and the concept of upward mobility.

It's also ironic that Matt got the same degrees basically I got at university. Both Matt and I got a Double Honours B.A. in English and History. He went on for a master's in library science, whereas I went on for a Master's in English. Matt took the more practical road, whereas I could not find a job with my Master's in English. I veered off to get a teaching degree and then wrote articles for a newspaper in Chilliwack, B.C.

It also surprised me that Matt ended up pretty well a home body sticking to one town, Tillsonburg. I've migrated through several provinces during my working career and even moved to France for a year with my wife to get a B.A. in French at the Université de Perpignan.

> Two roads diverged in a yellow wood,
> And sorry I could not travel both.
> -   *Robert Frost*

5

Reunion

I met Matt again when we were both old men, long in the tooth, you might say. There was a 40th reunion of St. Jerome's High School grads in 2005, I think. Matt was 1965; I was 1967, but I showed up anyway to his reunion. I'd already taken some web design courses at Mohawk College in night school and designed my own johnhartigphotography.com website. Actually, I'd created two websites, the other one being stjeromes66.com, as a tribute to the old high school.

We met at somebody's house in Kitchener. I brought a dozen DVD copies of the stjeromes66 site to give to Matt and friends. Several of the priests who had been our teachers were also invited. I remember Matt pointing to one of the priests: "He was a mean sonofabitch?" "No," I said. "He was okay in our class. A good teacher, but then maybe not so good with the bad kids."

I was speaking, of course, from my point of view. I was in the "browner" class, the 9A to 12A group. We were streamed. I can't remember what stream Matt was placed into, but streaming didn't mean anything. Many of those kids ended up execs, successful businesspeople with their own companies.

The priest he pointed out quit the priesthood. He'd gotten married and had two sons, and even wrote a book about fatherhood. I thought he made a good choice to get out of the priesthood because I always objected to the priestly vow to remain celibate. That to me, did not make sense. The rule caused the Catholic Church a barrel of grief.

Old alumni were pleased to get copies of my stjeromes66 website. It featured photos of teachers and students from those years in the 1960s. I don't know if the website has ever been passed on or preserved in somebody's computer because two decades have almost gone by since I last saw Matt. "Tempus fugit!" as Father Ruetz, the Latin teacher, used to say.

Matt must have been content living in the same place in Tillsonburg as a librarian. I'd been all over the globe by this time. At teacher's college in B.C., a news reporter for the Chilliwack Progress, an editor for "Grande Prairie This Week" in Alberta, an electrical apprentice at Grande Prairie College, a bible college student in Winnipeg, an exchange student in Perpignan France, a teacher again in Foleyet Ontario and finally, a wedding photographer and web designer trained at Mohawk College. None of those jobs suited me, except being editor of a paper. But then, the pay was peanuts. A writer cannot subsist on a byline.

When I finally got a computer, kicking and screaming that I would never get one, I embarked on a whole world of discovery in 2000, not only learning how to use one, but designing websites and learning the ins and outs of Photoshop.

In the decade that followed, I connected with Matt again and we intermittently e-mailed each other. That was also when I reconnected with Keith Kueneman, an old Vigilante friend, whom I had not seen for years. He and his wife, Mary-Pat, visited us in Vineland some years back in 2008. Keith and his wife are retired now and keep busy painting. Keith also is an avid fiddler. He never belonged to the St. Jerome's high school orchestra. He loves jamming, however, with friends. Their big love is "bluegrass." Keith and Mary-Pat live in Wasaga Beach, a three-hour drive from Tillsonburg.

There is nothing like a physical connection with an old friend. I'm glad Keith and his wife visited. I am also glad he can still play the fiddle. I guess I'm jealous a bit. I had to give up my violin playing back in 2008, the year my brother-in-law, Kenny, died. I tore the tendons in my shoulders lifting a heavy fan in my crawl space. Never do renovations yourself when you are getting on in years!

Thank goodness, I can still write and photograph. These are my creative outlets which keep me busy in my old age. I switched from wedding photography when I got injured to taking scenery photos with a small digital pocket camera. I get my fill of flower photos in the spring and colorful tree pictures in the autumn. These are my two favorite seasons.

6

The Pergola

[I summarized the scene at the Pergola in my own words, using some information from what Sean O'Sullivan wrote in the blog, Caring Bridge.]

People started trickling in about 10:00 o'clock, gathering around the pergola outside Matt's apartment building, the Oxford Estates. Matt lived on the third floor.

The superintendent for the Oxford Estates was kind enough to provide benches and chairs for people who wanted to show Matt support in this strange sort of "send-off." Matt came to the window to blow kisses to the crowd down below before the doctor took over for the procedure which had to inevitably follow.

It's all a shame that pain medication did not work for Matt. It's also ironic that Matt, a lifetime non-smoker, tried Cannabis to lessen his nausea, a drug which he hated. After 4 months of endurance, first with the operation to remove the tumor in his sinuses, and then having to put up with radiation treatments and pain medication which did not satisfactorily work. Matt finally said, "Enough." He wanted the hurting and the constant diarrhea to stop.

Yet, even as he stood by the open window on the third floor, he cracked one last joke for the crowd.

"I went ice fishing last month. 'Caught twenty pounds of ice and when I got home and tried to cook it, I nearly drowned."

This was a typical Matt joke, a real "groaner."

John Skinner, a tenant at the apartments, dressed in full Highland regalia, played Amazing Grace, so familiar to all of us, as Matt withdrew from the window.

I'm reminded of the saying by the Chief in the movie, Little Big Man, "It's a good day to die." The morning was sunny and warm.

John and Liz Monroe, close neighbors, served champagne and orange juice to toast Matt after he departed this world.

Matt was an ordinary man and yet so extraordinary in many ways.

His son, Andrew, traced Matt's achievements throughout his life by writing this eulogy on the man who led a life well-lived.

*****

Matthew G. Scholtz
April 6, 1946 - June 19, 2023
Husband, father, always curious about life.

He came into this world naturally, but left it on his own terms, on June 19, 2023, after a four-month, long suffering battle with complications from cancer.

Matthew Scholtz is especially pleased to make his final exit currently, to avoid the next 18 months of crazy, unprincipled, and ugly American politics.

Born in Czechoslovakia on April 6, 1946, Matt lived in Germany until his family immigrated to Kitchener, Ontario in April 1951. After graduating from St. Jerome's High School in Kitchener, he attended the University of Western

Ontario, where he earned an Honours B.A. in History and English, followed by an M.A. in Library Science.

In August 1970, he was appointed Chief Librarian of the Tillsonburg Public Library, a position he held until his retirement in September 2010. He founded and became the first chairperson of the Association of Small Public Libraries of Ontario (1980) and served on many area and provincial library committees.

In his early tenure at the library, he was given a professional opportunity: design and manage a new Public Library. The new building opened in June 1975, but without his presence at the official opening ceremonies. Exhausted by the final preparations, he wound up in the hospital with pneumonia.

In 1984, he edited and provided photographs for "Tillsonburg: A History, 1825-1982", which was co-authored by J.I. Cooper and John Armstrong. A decade later, he wrote "Tillsonburg Diary: A Chronological History 1824-1994", based on a monograph by Anna M. Bailey. His last book, "Tillsonburg Album: A Photographic History," was published in 2014.

Aside from being Library C.E.O., he served as Executive Secretary of the Tillsonburg Chamber of Commerce (1977 - 2010), and as a freelance correspondent for the London Free Press (1976 – 1990). For the Tillsonburg News, he wrote two weekly columns over 40 years, one dealing with library issues and the other with local history.

He was active in Theatre Tillsonburg, on and off stage, as well as administratively as long-term, long-suffering treasurer of the Theatre Board.

There was nothing that pleased him more than to make people smile by telling a joke. It was nothing unusual for him to approach a stranger and ask," Did you hear about the fire in London? Yes, a shoe factory burned down. 2,000 soles were lost! And it was started by a heel!" Or: "If at first you don't succeed, I do not recommend skydiving for you." And everyone's favourite: "A friend suggested I put horse manure on my strawberries. Tried it. Didn't like it. Went back to whipping cream." He always kept his jokes short. That was because if you did not like the first one, he had another for you.

Matt believed that if you can make a person smile, you will not change the world, but you will change theirs.
In September 2010, he retired from the Tillsonburg Library and befriended a student he met in a library correspondence course he had been teaching online since 1995. In October 2011, he married that student, Leni Kraska. Together, they built new lives together, first in Bainsville, Ontario and after 2013, in Tillsonburg.

In his retirement, he enjoyed helping people compose their life story, but his special joy was book repairing. Matt loved to restore books for those who valued them, attracting clients from across Canada.

Matt wanted to recognize the important contribution made by Sue Rodrigues. Some thirty years ago, she failed to win her court case for death with dignity, but she

ignited a conversation on that issue that led to our current legislation enabling it. Suffering Canadians owe her a lot.
Predeceased by his wife, Betty (1941 – 2010). He is survived by his wife, Leni (Magdalena) and sons, Stephen (Jessica) and Andrew (Erin). Also survived by stepsons (aka bonus sons) James (Micheline), Peter (Kelly), and Matthew (Shasta). And special brother-in-law Joe Virag.

Cremation has taken place. There was no funeral or visitation. A Celebration of Life will be held at a date, to be announced.

Thank-you so much for all your love and prayers.
- Andrew Scholtz

7
MAiD

When I was in religion class in grade 9, I remember the priest telling us that if you commit suicide, you committed a mortal sin and that you were condemned to hell.

Matt would have had the same priests I had as teachers in our all-boys Catholic school, St. Jerome's in Kitchener. Even then, I had a hard time swallowing what those priests said.

I remember thinking, how does this priest know? How does he know the suffering a person goes through to make a person desperate enough to take one's life? Isn't a professionally monitored procedure, one without pain, better than a shotgun?

MAiD became legal in Canada in June 2016, with the passage of Bill C-14, which amended the Criminal Code and other federal acts with respect to medical assistance in dying.

I suppose well-to-do, rich countries like Canada and the United States consider themselves progressive in their thinking by giving their terminally ill patients a painless option to end life by Medical Assistance in Dying.

MAiD has been called by other names, like mercy killing, assisted suicide and euthanasia.

Canada is ranked third in the world for having the most well-developed public health care system. Yet, in the past few decades, the system has failed, clogged by huge wait times and hallway healthcare. Money seems to be behind this failure. The disbursement of funds from the federal coffers to the provinces and territories has failed. While the federal government promises huge money for the support of the war effort in Ukraine against Russia, it does not have enough money to bolster up its own infrastructure for hospital workers and healthcare in Canada.

Among the top 10 laudable healthcare systems are Scandinavian countries like Sweden, Norway, also the Netherlands and Finland. Their healthcare is paid for by tax money, plus nominal user fees. The United States, as a supposed rich civilized country, does not even rate in the top 10. Even a little country like Costa Rica is ranked 36th in the world by the World Health Organization, above the United States, Cuba, and New Zealand. The United Nations placed Costa Rica within the top 20 in the world. Costa Rica has free public healthcare, but only for citizens who are in most financial need. They don't have a military, the money going to the healthcare of its people, a clever choice in priorities.

Whether healthcare is provided by taxation, private insurance, whether healthcare is considered universal or private, it all comes back to money!

To keep someone alive who is terminally ill, for as long as possible, costs money. There are, of course, a whole raft of legal and moral issues involved in the option of medically assisted dying. The medical profession is aware of the sensitive choice of words. Dying, for instance, sounds better than the blunt word, death. The word euthanasia is a fancy word that many people still do not know, so the reality of death is obfuscated by fancy terminology.

Since MAiD was legalized in 2016 in Canada, euthanasia is ranked Canada's sixth leading cause of death.

The movement to adopt this option has become so swift in some countries that the United Nations "special rapporteur on Rights of persons with Disabilities" has raised concerns. Churches tend to stay away from the controversy, refraining to say anything as a whole, but restricting itself to a "nonjudgmental provider of pastoral care" for the individual who is about to undergo the procedure.

It seems alright according to the Supreme Court's decision in Canada in 2015 that euthanasia has become a human right, but only under specific circumstances:

> The person requesting it must have a "grievous and irremediable medical condition" that is incurable, irreversible, and involves unendurable suffering, in which "natural death has become reasonably foreseeable." Furthermore, consent at the time of the person's death was required, as was a ten-day waiting period. Children and those whose only diagnosis was mental illness were not eligible.
> ["Plough Quarterly", article by Benjamin Crosby]

Disability rights groups hated the new law seeing themselves as victims of a kind of genocide of their kind.

It did not take long for this law to be criticized as too constraining by other groups who wanted the eligibility to be broadened. They wanted Canada to be more progressive. Parliament changed the law, introducing C-7, which removed constraints.

Euthanasia became available for those nowhere near dying, including people who suffered from an incurable combination of physical and mental ills. The curve rose dramatically from 1,018 deaths in 2016 to 10,064 deaths in 2021.

Assisted suicide was made available in some states in the United States, involving a different procedure than MAiD where the patient takes an active part in "the act." With euthanasia a doctor injects a needle directly. With the other method, in some states, the patient has to swallow a lethal drug by his or her own hand.

In terms of broadening the eligibility for MAiD, "progressive" groups are lobbying for making incurable depression and other mental disorders eligible. In terms of the original law, nothing is written in stone.

MAiD is obviously cost effective for the government. Would it be less needed, if the system would work faster, if we had small wait times, and if specialists were available within a reasonable time. The question is obviously, yes. If the system were less broken, patients in a crisis could lead a better quality of life, even with handicaps. Again, all this comes back to two things: healthcare manpower and money.

8
Broadening Eligibility

Euphemisms are words that make the reality of dire situations seem not so bad. MAiD is marketed as a procedure to end one's life in a gentle and nonthreatening manner.

You can actually find "death doulas" who comfort MAiD patients, their families, and friends, with soothing words telling the patient to dress warmly and hydrate, "encouraging the bereaved to process the experience through grounding themselves in their bodies or expressing themselves through dance." [Plough Quarterly, article by Benjamin Crosby]

Death doulas are paid privately by the family on a scale of time and expenses spent. Nothing is free in this life.

Journalist, Benjamin Crosby, sees medical assistance in dying as "cloaked in anesthetizing therapeutic language."

The champions for MAiD see patients freeing themselves from the dependence on diapers, of having to live with diarrhea and drooling. These proponents demand that patients have the right to end their lives with dignity. They should not be stuck with a poor quality of life.

There doesn't seem to be a choice for some people within our system. Some patients pursue the process because the support services they need in our society are too slow where applications for help seem to go in circles or get stuck in bureaucracy. They can't live a decent life, while they are forced to fill out applications for help and wait. Where is the money to free our clogged system?

With no choice, even some health care providers are inclined to push the idea that "we do have a way out of your pain."

Journalist, Benjamin Crosby, cited an example of Sophia, a 51-year-old woman who suffered from MCS, multiple chemical sensitivities. She could not find an apartment that met her needs.

"The government sees me as expendable trash, a complainer, useless, and a pain in the ass," she said in a video a few days before she was killed via MAiD in February 2022. [Plough Quarterly, article by Benjamin Crosby]

"Kat," a woman in her late thirties with a genetic disorder, cannot afford her treatments. "I feel like I'm falling through the cracks, so if I'm not able to access health care am I then able to access death care?" she told CTV News. She has been approved for what she calls an "open invitation" to go through with MAiD at any time. [Plough Quarterly, article by Benjamin Crosby]

Alan, a sixty-one-year-old man, was hospitalized for his wish to commit suicide and, within a month, applied for MAiD. He was killed over the objections of family members and his primary medical provider, who alleged that he did not understand MAiD and was coerced into it by hospital staff. The only condition listed on his MAiD application was hearing loss. [Plough Quarterly, article by Benjamin Crosby]

Sathya, a forty-four-year-old woman who suffered from ALS but for whom natural death was not imminent, was killed via MAiD because she could not access home care. "Ultimately, it was not a genetic disease which took me out, it was a system," she wrote shortly before her death in October 2022. [Plough Quarterly, article by Benjamin Crosby]

It is an important function of a reporter, like Benjamin Crosby, to bring out the shortcomings, if not the wrong doings of the system, to the public. We brag about our gentler and kinder society in Canada, and yet there is a "grievous betrayal", as Mr. Crosby calls it, when MAiD is considered a solution to poverty and disability.

Perhaps, my friend's choice was right for himself. I cannot judge his pain and his medical and moral decision, but as a writer, I need to speak out about these issues in my research about the system which ended my friend's life. Who knows if his quality of life could have been bearable had the system not failed him in other ways, like wait times, and quick access to pain management.

Like the reporter, Benjamin Crosby, I too, along with Matt, were immigrants to Canada. We've thrived here in the education system and also benefited from Canada's healthcare in the early years. But one must question in which direction our adopted country is going.

Will the next broadening of parameters be simply "quality of life" which could mean anything? That is so far removed from the terminally ill definition of 2016.

I wonder about the moral lines when we make someone eligible for medical assistance in dying. I can understand the qualms that people with disabilities have, those in wheelchairs or those dealing with a long-acting disease like MS or ASL. If a person's problem is housing or homecare, should that not be taken care of first?

Perhaps, a quadriplegic in a wheelchair, who cannot get proper housing, might think that the system in Canada is approaching what Hitler in Nazi Germany wanted, after all, getting rid of burdens in society.

I do understand someone in chronic pain, every second of the day, wanting to have a way out. I have torn tendons in my shoulders and a torn meniscus in my knee. I take half an Oxycocet every 4 hours. I had to wait a year to get into a pain management clinic. Now, I can live with my pain and am producing a book every 6 months and publishing them on Amazon. I do not make any money out of my projects. I donate my books and novels to seniors' homes around the Niagara Peninsula.

I live with a purpose, thankfully finding a doctor, even if it took a year, to manage my pain. But if it were not for pain management and finally getting in, I do not know what I would do. I will not judge my friend Matt and do not know all the circumstances. Yes, I can understand the people who take the option of medical assistance in dying. I've sort of touched on those thoughts myself. Benjamin Crosby cited someone in his article about what that person felt about their journey in pain that they'd want to escape:

> I do not want to linger in pain, waiting for death to come. I do not want my family and loved ones to watch me suffer to the bitter end. I do not want them to be haunted by memories of a slow, painful death. Daily my dignity is being eroded. I am ready to go through that final door. *I give thanks that I have still the ability to choose, but I realize this window of lucid opportunity may very soon be closed* [emphasis original].

9
Opposing MAiD

Journalist, Benjamin Crosby is openly against MAiD not expanding its mandate to euthanize more people with chronic conditions. He writes for the Christian magazine, "Plough Quarterly." He is disappointed in churches taking a neutral stance on the issue, not to rock the political boat, but to give only specific comfort to the individual seeking MAiD. He stands with the disabled community who see their right to life threatened by a government which can't find the funds for supporting them.

There are wider issues than putting the terminally ill and chronic sufferers of pain out of their misery.

The disabled fear for their lives and rightly so if help is not there. So do the intellectually disabled. Crosby sees Christians taking a positive stand to oppose the "negative stereotypes about people with disabilities." Society sees them as suffering, in need of state-regulated assistance to end their lives. [Plough Quarterly, article by Benjamin Crosby]

We must not embrace the feeling that some persons' lives are not worth living. That is a dangerous and slippery slope.

Of course, such an impression may not apply to my friend Matt's decision. He ended his continual pain with a decision that was right for him. But knowing him as the second person, whom I personally knew, who used MAiD to end a poor quality of life, I am moved to write this book and ask some serious questions about the current money problems in Canada's healthcare system and also in the rising use of MAiD. We need to find the funds somehow to create positive stories about how the system helped people who can live with disabilities, frailty, and suffering, provided they are properly funded and taken care of.

I often think that our politicians are stuck in the mud, arguing from party affiliations, instead of making decisions about what is good for the whole country and good for its citizens. MAiD, I'm sure, has served a great purpose in our society giving dignity to those who are indeed terminally ill and suffering from intense chronic pain day after day. But we must ask, where do we, as a society, draw the line on the use of MAiD and our regard for the "sacredness" of life, if we regard life as "sacred," even if we don't believe in a God.

It is interesting that googling whether physicians in Canada still swear by the Hippocratic Oath, I found this: that the Hippocratic Oath, which is still administered in many but not all medical schools, omits any reference to a moral obligation on the part of physicians to be honest with their patients. The Hippocratic Oath has been replaced new words and by new codes of ethics, such as the Declaration of Geneva and that of the Canadian Medical Association, which forgoes many things in the original ancient Oath. This means, in short, that modern doctors do not swear "First, do no harm" and also do not swear "to preserve life."

10

The Little Things

Our morning chores left some impressions in my mind. Matt is no longer bothered either by the good or the bad of such chores, nor the worries of daily living.

My Lifelabs blood test went quickly. I always pre-book online. When we went to Edible Options afterwards, I got out of the car to do my cross over foot exercise with a little bending. That was better than sitting in the car. I soaked in the sunshine while my wife was in the store. It felt so good. I wore socks today, since my big toes broke out in red with crazy itchiness due to the radiation from the sun. A new sensitivity to deal with! Oh well. I was glad to get home to soak my feet in cold water. What a relief.

We dropped off at Walmart to get a few bananas and also the Butterballs hot dogs that I like for when we do a wienie roast in the backyard. The fire ban down here has been lifted. We will have to phone Fair Havens in the Muskoka area to see if they still have their fire ban on. Our stay at the trailer will be sporadic that summer since Marilyn and Jerry often use the other resort run by their son and his wife's relatives who own Shalom by the Lake outside of Minden.

I told my wife that she could get a handful of Bridge Mix at the Bulk Barn if she wanted. That used to be our treat driving home from grocery shopping, but now, I have cut myself off sweets to keep my Triglycerides down.

While Marjorie was in the Bulk Barn, I decided to do walking laps around the car. The sun warmed my shoulders, a nice feeling. Matt has been dead for two days now. I thought of him as I gazed up at the wonderful blue sky. I am grateful for the little things in my life that I can feel, see, and touch.

When Marjorie finally came out of the store, I fished for the first handful of chocolate treats to give her, before she put the car into Drive. We passed our usual homeless man at the corner of 4th Avenue by the lights. He had a big placard which read, *Homeless and Hungry*. Marjorie commented that if he had been near the Superstore, she would have bought him a meal. She'd done that before.

The first thing I did when we got home was for me to put my feet into 4 inches of cold water in the bathtub. I imagined that my feet went, ZZZSSSSt, with steam coming off them. They felt so hot and itchy. I think the vivid red on my toes is subsiding. We ate our Quinoa salads on our TV trays, listening to the news. Barrie has a new law. The town will levy a fine on anybody who gives food to the homeless a hefty $100,000 fine! A Barrie grandmother is protesting this ban. I suppose if Barrie gets rid of their homeless people and makes them move either to Newmarket or to Toronto, then Barrie can brag that they've solved their homeless problem. They can advertise Barrie as a healthy community where middle-class families would want to move to.

The Barrie grandmother says that such a ban is against human rights. I agree with her, thinking about that homeless guy at the lights on 4th Avenue, holding out his placard for handouts. I don't remember things like this when I was a boy in Canada.

Barrie has since backed off from a law against homeless people begging for handouts, which discriminates against them. Who wants bad publicity?

I wonder if Matt's little town of Tillsonburg, population 18,000, has a homeless problem?

The Avondale United Church in Tillsonburg offered its basement as a shelter for the homeless throughout the winter because the homeless problem in this little town was noticeably growing. Ontario mayors say that the homeless are less visible in small, rural towns. Apparently, the problem has grown into a visible problem since the Pandemic and the rising cost of housing, which in Toronto is ridiculous.

As a librarian, I wonder if Matt saw more homeless "types" coming into the library to bide their time there, especially in the cold winter months. I know Vineland's Rittenhouse library had no homeless "types" coming in to stay warm. Homeless people, who actually looked homeless, frequented Tim Horton's instead, off the QEW and off 4th Avenue, where they could nurse a coffee way past the 20-minute time limit. Tim Horton's seems to have a more flexible rule about the loitering time limit than Starbucks.

I phoned a friend who is in charge of a greenhouse in the Niagara Region and asked if any of the migrant workers there could use a good used bike. Migrants use old bicycles all the time in Vineland doing their grocery shopping at Foodland. "Sure," said my friend. We just need to arrange a time for the pickup.

Unions like OPSEU have taken Ford's provincial government to court demanding to repeal Bill 124, which restricts the wage increase to 1% while inflation goes up 11%. Ford is clearly anti-union and anti-rights to negotiate new contracts.

These are hard times! Stephen Foster wrote about hard times way back in 1854. Nothing has changed.

Let us pause in life's pleasures.
and count its many tears,
While we all sup sorrow with the poor.
There's a song that will linger forever in our ears,
Oh, hard times, come again no more.

Well, my wife has gone to the Ladies' Strawberry Social at the church while I write this. We've finished our Quinoa lunch and turned the TV off. Nothing but bad news on TV anyway. The submersible which had 5 people in it for sightseeing of the sunken Titanic is still missing. They have oxygen, it is estimated, until tomorrow morning. How do they feel, knowing that they will die possibly tomorrow. Passengers include Stockton Rush, the executive for OceanGate Expeditions, Hamish Harding, a British businessman and explorer, Paul-Henri Nargeolet, a French maritime expert, and Shahzada and Suleman Dawood, a father and son, British/Pakistani billionaires from textiles and fertilizer manufacturing. All their apparent health and their wealth cannot save them, unless by chance, the rescuing crew comes upon them.

In the meantime, the war in Ukraine rages on. Bodies are shot to pieces and families destroyed with the missiles which hit apartment buildings. Death, so senseless, when Matt could have used a healthy body to stick around for another decade or so for his wife and kids.

My wife is still at the Ladies' Strawberry Social. It's a woman's thing; no men allowed. I will take the basketball, ride my e-bike to the church and bounce the ball for a bit. I will not wear my Crocs without my socks. Afterwards, it will be time for a cold-water footbath again.

11

A Kinder Society

UPDATE:

Thursday was the last day for that submersible when its oxygen ran out. After days of searching, rescue crews found debris. What a sad ending for rich explorers who wanted to say they'd been down to the debris of the Titanic which originally lost 1,500 lives after hitting an iceberg back in 1912. Not even a billionaire was safe from death when Mother Nature crushed the submersible in the depth of the ocean floor. Bodies have not been recovered. It's ironic that these business tycoons have added their own bodies now to that of the Titanic, where they intended to use the 1912 tragedy as a money-making tourist attraction.

Our planet that floats in outer space is like the submersible. We are suspended in the depth of deep space, protected by the shell of our atmosphere. Our oxygen could be running out as we neglect climate change and continue to pollute the atmosphere.

We've come a long way along our tumultuous and violent history of wars and racial hatreds. What can we brag about, as we send rockets into deep space to explore other planets? We have the power to blow up the planet and leave earth's debris sadly floating in pieces in deep space. Who will rescue us?

I am always sorry to hear distressing news on TV and I thank God that bad things like a world war have not happened again. No matter how much money those explorers in the submersible had, they were not saved by their wealth. I am sad for their families and imagine the fear those 5 people must have experienced in the last seconds of their lives before the submersible imploded. I suppose nothing is guaranteed, certainly not life.

*****

SQUEAKY WHEEL:

The movement towards euthanasia in Canada has been long and arduous, overcoming legal challenges which frustrated sick people who were in terrible pain and who knew that their inevitable end was near. Why prolong the pain and the terrible quality of life?

Weak voices throughout Canada have now been heard because of their persistence and because of their heart-wrenching suffering.

The federal government decriminalized attempted suicide in 1972 and the legal right to turn down medical treatment emerged at around the same time, as technological advances in medicine allowed doctors to keep patients alive longer. Not everybody, however, wanted to live longer!

In the 1970s, a series of court cases won a mentally competent person the right to refuse medical intervention.

The debate over patient autonomy today centers on issues of active euthanasia and assisted suicide, as patients who live in chronic, intense pain or with a degenerative or terminal illness such as multiple sclerosis, AIDS or Alzheimer's disease, fight for the right to choose to die.

*****

HISTORY ON RIGHT TO DIE:
*Resource: CBC News · **Posted: Feb 05, 2015**

1991: The Right to Die Society is founded in Canada in Victoria, B.C. to help guide those who need assistance in dying and to lobby for the legalization of assisted suicide.

December 1992: MP Svend Robinson, the New Democratic Party MP from Burnaby-Kingsway in B.C., introduces a private member's bill, C-385, "to allow for physician-assisted suicide upon the request of a terminally ill person." The closing of Parliament prevents the bill from coming forward for debate.

1992: Sue Rodriguez begins her fight to overturn the law banning doctor-assisted death in Canada.

Sept. 30, 1993: The Supreme Court of Canada, in a 5-4 decision, dismisses the appeal of Sue Rodriguez, who has ALS (a.k.a. Lou Gehrig's disease) and wants a physician to help her die. The decision includes concerns about potential abuse and the difficulty of creating appropriate safeguards.

February 1994: Sue Rodriguez, assisted by an unknown doctor, dies in her home in Victoria. MP Svend Robinson witnesses her death. In 1992, ALS patient Sue Rodriguez began her fight to overturn the law banning doctor-assisted death in Canada. That culminated in a landmark 1993 Supreme Court of Canada decision dismissing her case. Rodriguez died in 1994.

1998: Maurice Généreux becomes the first doctor to be sentenced under the law banning physician-assisted death. The Quebec doctor received a jail term of two years less a day and three years' probation in 1998 for prescribing sleeping pills to two men with AIDS who were depressed but not terminally ill. One of the men survived and later launched a civil suit against Généreux.

June 2007: Dr. Ramesh Kumar Sharm of Vernon, B.C. is given a conditional sentence of two years less a day and has his physician's license revoked after prescribing a lethal dose of drugs for a 93-year-old patient.

December 2008: A Quebec jury acquits Stephan Dufour on a single charge of assisted suicide. Dufour had admitted to installing in a closet a rope, chain, and dog collar that his uncle, Chantal Maltais, used to kill himself in September 2006. Dufour was the first Canadian ever to stand trial by jury for assisted suicide.

May 2009: MP Francine Lalonde introduces a private members' bill for the second time "to allow a medical practitioner, subject to certain conditions, to aid a person who is experiencing severe physical or mental pain without any prospect of relief or is suffering from a terminal illness to die with dignity once the person has expressed his or her free and informed consent to die." It does not pass, and the MP soon resigns. Lalonde dies of bone cancer in January 2014.

June 2012: B.C. Supreme Court Justice Lynn Smith, in a case that includes ALS patient Gloria Taylor, declares Canada's laws against physician assisted suicide unconstitutional because they discriminate against the physically disabled. In a 395-page ruling, Smith noted suicide itself is not illegal, and therefore the law against assisted suicide contravenes Section 15 of the Charter, which guarantees equality, because it denies physically disabled people like Taylor the same rights as able-bodied people who can take their own lives. Smith also said the law deprives both people like Taylor and those who try to help them of the right to life and liberty guaranteed under Section 7 of the charter. The federal government appeals the ruling to the B.C. Court of Appeals.

October 2012: Gloria Taylor, the ALS patient who spearheaded the movement to change Canada's right-to-die laws, dies from an infection.

February 6, 2015: The Supreme Court of Canada unanimously overturns a legal ban on doctor-assisted suicide, ruling the law should be amended to allow doctors to help in specific situations.

January 6, 2015: The Supreme Court of Canada hears an appeal from the B.C. Civil Liberties Association seeking to overturn the legal ban on doctor-assisted dying.

August 2014: Gillian Bennett, a B.C. woman diagnosed with dementia three years ago, kills herself by ingesting drugs. Before her death, she posted on her blog that she feared she would become a burden on her family and did not want to spend "an indefinite number of years of being a vegetable in a hospital setting." Bennett also hoped to reopen the debate about assisted suicide.

June 2014: The National Assembly in Quebec passes Bill 52, known as "the dying with dignity law", allowing terminally ill patients to have medical aid in dying. The bill follows Europe's lead by extending the law's reach to those experiencing "unbearable suffering," but who may not be within months of dying.

March 2014: Winnipeg Tory MP Steven Fletcher introduces two private members bills. One allows doctors to help people end their lives under certain restricted circumstances, including the individual must be of "sound mind" with "an illness, a disease or disability (including disability arising from traumatic injury) that causes physical or psychological suffering that is intolerable to that person and that cannot be alleviated by any medical treatment acceptable to that person." The other bill proposes a commission to monitor the system.

January 6, 2015: The Supreme Court of Canada hears an appeal from the B.C. Civil Liberties Association seeking to overturn the legal ban on doctor-assisted dying.

February 6, 2015: The Supreme Court of Canada unanimously overturns a legal ban on doctor-assisted suicide, ruling the law should be amended to allow doctors to help in specific situations.

May 23, 2017: Robyn Moro, 65, who has Parkinson's disease is the latest person to join the legal fight to overturn limitations preventing those whose deaths are not "reasonably foreseeable" from having medically assisted death. [CBC News article posted May 23, 2023]

The controversial requirement was part of federal legislation in June 2016. The argument went to the

Supreme Court. Moro confessed, "I have so much pain every day and I know my Parkinson's will only continue to get worse." She said, "the law is forcing me to suffer."

Julia Lamb, 25, who suffers from spinal muscular atrophy joined the fight to lift restrictions on people who suffer from "grievous" but not terminal illnesses.

Jay Aubrey, lawyer, said, "People who experience horrific, irremediable suffering, but whose death is not yet reasonably foreseeable, are left with two choices — to continue to suffer intolerably against their will, or to turn to non-medical ways of ending their life, such as starvation and dehydration." He added, "This is a cruel choice. Surely we have more compassion than to leave people to suffer and die in this way."

12
Caring Bridge

Caring Bridge is a non-profit website which over 25 years has supported sick people who do not wish to go through health journeys alone. It gives friends and relatives access to the entries which are posted by someone sick or recovering, so that time consuming individual e-mails do not have to be mailed out. Friends and relatives can relay messages of love and support through Caring Bridge in an efficient way.

Matt's Story was started on Caring Bridge on January 10, 2023.

When I got the notice from Matt's family about Caring Bridge, I jumped at the chance to express my concern and encouragement for every time Matt, or his sons, posted something.

Matt posted the sad news of his decision to use MAiD, on Thursday June 15, 2023: "My recovery from January's cancer surgery went well for a time. Then it didn't." This chapter follows the first few months of hopefulness and well wishing from his friends. Then comes a later chapter which outlines the reaction of his friends when Matt posted the sad news that he decided to die.

So, in the first hopeful months, starting on January 23, 2023, his son, Stephen, wrote: "Leni was complaining about how her coffee wasn't ready in the morning, and Dad didn't train me well for his absence. Looks like that was all part of Dad's plan. :) "Did not train, and therefore you need to appreciate me!"

Matt Scholtz carried his sense of humor and his addiction to silly jokes into any dire circumstances. As a librarian, he had an encyclopedic memory for jokes, most of them groaners. He was a genius with groaners!

Stephen posted a journal entry for his dad on January 25, 2023, where he described how Leni and he saw Matt off to his operation that morning, in the dark, at 4:00 a.m. Even at that ungodly hour, Matt's humor was evident. When he was asked if he had any allergies, he quickly said, "No, just work!"

It's hard to believe that an operation could last up to 10 hours. However, an operation on the face, on the sinuses to remove a tumor, was extremely intricate. The plan was to visit him the next day, probably in the afternoon.

Stephen tried to emulate Matt's usual ending in the Blog with a joke. This one was about a tip: Don't make any jokes about German sausage...they're the wurst.

My personal response on Caring Bridge was, "Thanks, Stephen. Marjorie and I are still praying. This, I'm sure, took a lot out of Matt. "

Matt had to use a white board on January 27, when he came out of anesthesia, using a red marker to scribble things like: "Pain terrible yesterday, today." He added, "We need to develop shorthand for this." Matt also wrote, "Right now, I would love a big Mac!!!"

Matt ended the white board messages with the drawing of a heart and a little U in it, for I love you to Leni. Stephen's comment was that his dad was charming Leni.

By January 28, the nurses were getting Matt up to sit. Walking was limited and of course dangerous. Matt tried to help his nurses with the bit of walking, but it was complicated because of all the tubes.

Things were sporadic and slow on postings as Matt slowly, very slowly got better. His cheek was swollen and hurt.

His son, Andrew Scholtz made a significant entry on May 16 telling friends and relatives just that. "This is going to take a long, long time." Tube feedings were the order of the day, not as filling as a Big Mac! Matt already lost the hearing in his left ear. Dr. MacNeill suggested a consultation within 3 months, which would mean August. However, sadly Matt never made it to August.

I am not sure if Matt dictated his entry, but he mentioned costly dental work. He also mentioned for the first time, "Honestly friends, if I had known ahead of time just what I was in for, well, I would have declined treatment and chosen MAiD (as a friend recently did)."

Matt described not only living one day at a time during the past 4 months, but "surviving one minute at a time." He confessed that he and Leni had not discussed MAiD at that time, so the topic was not discussed. They had decided though, that there would be no third cancer journey. Matt said that the cure is really worse than the disease.

I was amused that he quoted one of my favorite rock groups, Trooper: "We're here for a good time; not a long time. So, have a good time; the sun can't shine every day."

13

Rallying Cries

His friends rallied in response to the sad turn of events. Matt was supposed to get better, albeit slowly, with the operation and with radiation treatments. When Matt first mentioned MAiD, his friends were taken aback.

On May 16, I wrote: "Forget MAiD now, Matt. You are getting better slowly, it's going to take a long, long time yet, but you are over the hump."

Lorna Graham wrote: "What you have endured! I appreciate your honest account of what this experience has been like for you and Leni. It's so hard to make an informed decision about treatment because we really don't have all the information until we live through it, do we? Thanks for sharing, Matt, and hang in there!"

On May 17, Randy Ray wrote: "Yikes. Be strong and make the decision that is best for you. I support whatever you feel is best for your life going forward. And the lives of those around you. I love you buddy!"

Neave Greig wrote: "to heck with MAiD Matt, you have it MADE with your indomitable spirit, courage, Leni, and your kids. You have come so far, so persevere and keep your eyes on life, family, love, friends, and the future. We have a lot of good times and games yet to share. We can't imagine life without you so keep on going one day at a time. Selfish on our part but so what, we don't have enough friends to let you go. Lots of love from me and Ted."

Matt showed immense courage throughout the radiation treatment in March with that mask he had to wear. The technician, Kristopher, was very helpful and encouraging.

After Matt's sad decision, Caring Bridge recorded a total of 4,578 visits over 4 months.

*****

I e-mailed Keith Kueneman directly in June, not knowing if he kept up with what was happening with Matt. I wrote this:

> I was surprised how quickly the process with MAiD went. Procedure applied at 11 a.m. on Monday and cremated the same day. I did not realize how badly the side effects of Matt's cancer treatment were affecting him. I decided to write a novella about our experiences as kids at Victoria Park. How I met Matt and John and what fun we had in those days. Also, my ideas on Canada's progressive MAiD program. Good or bad? Are you going to go to his celebration of life once a date has been set?

Keith promptly replied:

> June20, 2023
> Hi John,
>
> I checked in with Matt on June 13 by email when I hadn't heard from him and when there were no more postings on Caring Bridge. He replied that he had signed up for MAiD (sorry I don't know what day he signed up).

Earlier, he said the pain was unbearable every second of the day. I don't believe you can just sign up, and actually have it done on the same day. There must be protocol and doctor discussions etc. before you can have it administered before it is determined that it can be a "go"?

I cannot imagine what he went through. I cringe and cry for him and cannot get him out of my mind at the moment. We have been friends since he arrived on Courtland Ave around 1952. I will miss him as will you. I don't think I will attend the celebration of life but will decide later. Long way from Wasaga Beach with a heavy heart.

Best to you and Marjorie.
Keith & Mary-Pat

Later that afternoon, I e-mailed Keith about the fact that Matt was the second person I knew who used MAiD. I felt that the approval went fast, almost too fast, probably within a week or two. "I think this will be the trend of the future in Canada. Getting psychiatric care, a pain clinic or surgery is very slow in this country. I am disappointed with the system." Keith echoed my sentiment:

June 20, 2023, at 1:27 PM
Hi John,

The whole government system sucks. Governments have poor talent in all parties, so they react, then have studies, then they increase taxes, then leave the garbage for the next government with more debt when they get voted out.

Unfortunately, all parties do not agree on agendas and do not work together. When the new government takes over, it works on their agenda, and nothing moves forward. It's sad. Trudeau is a huge disappointment. Only thing he knows, is how to waste taxpayers $$. Time for a change, but to what??

For Matt, losing left ear hearing, one nostril not working, not being able to eat with swollen cheeks, being fed with a tube, along with extreme pain and discomfort, I am happy he finally has relief. Rest in Peace Matthew!

Keith

14
Condolences

After Matt posted his sad decision to use MAiD on Thursday June 15, it was a black day in June for sure.

A whole bunch of responses flooded in, mostly sympathy, understanding, and also respecting Matt's decision for his final exit. People expressed condolences galore.

There were so many immediate responses on Thursday, June 15. I selected a few which represented the general burst of emotion and sympathy. Of course, I could not include all the friends who expressed their sentiments on Caring Bridge to keep this chapter to a reasonable length.

June 15: Della Hill wrote a touching tribute of what Matt had meant to them:

> Matt:
> We are very saddened to hear that you have endured so much suffering and that this is your decision. We can only imagine how hard this journey has been for you and your loved ones. This must be a very difficult decision for you, and we know you would have poured your energy into deciding this was the best option for you. We will miss you; you are a very special person.
> I want to thank you for so many things, here are a few:

- For being the welcoming neighbour on the day we moved in across the hall from you. For bringing over appreciated beer and cakes. Leni is a wonderful baker.
- For catching me with all your witty jokes, the one that I loved the most was the one about the fire in a shoe factory. You got me good on that one.
- For having us over to chat, play cards and enjoy at G&T
- For your wonderful suggestions on things to participate in. Theatre, choir, cards, libraries in the area.
- For leaving Chocolates on the shelf outside our door whenever the grandkids were visiting.
- For stopping by with chocolate liqueurs during the holidays.
- For taking us to your friend's hobby farm so our youngest granddaughter could meet the goats.
- For engaging us with your charm and companionship numerous evenings under the pergola.
- For buzzing me into the building when I forgot my keys and phone.
- But most of all for being the extra special man that you are taking us into your circle of friendship. Jim and I feel eternally grateful and privileged to have met you and been able to spend time with you over the past two years. You will forever be in our hearts and on our minds.

Rest easy,
Della and Jim

Rayburn Lansdell, the satellite director of Youth Unlimited: "Thank you, Matt, for including me in your personal and intimate message regarding your decision. After visiting briefly with you last week and hearing about your doctors' appointments this news doesn't come as a surprise, but I didn't realize the process would move along so quickly.

I pray that you will be drawn into the loving care of our heavenly FATHER, even though you have felt at times, and even now are feeling, that He has been absent on this very difficult journey you've been on. May you find comfort in knowing HIS love for you, that eternity awaits where there is no pain, no sorrow, no tears, and that you will be welcomed into heaven because of the saving sacrifice of Jesus where he awaits to present you to God. May your faith in Jesus carry you home.

Instead of goodbye, I will say, see you later ...because of Jesus."

Suzanne Renken: "Oh Matt, I can't stop crying. You've been so brave.
Thank you for being so open with all of us throughout your journey and for being the man you are. You were a wonderful champion when I worked alongside you during my first early years in my job with the Chamber - while you were still our Town's Librarian. I still walk into the library and think of you.

God Bless You,"

*****

I responded a few days later on Monday, June 19, the very day that Matt breathed his last. I did not know what to say. I finally wrote:

> Matt and I have a parallel history. My family came to Kitchener in 1954 from Austria. I was only two years behind him at St. Jerome's High. The school gave me a chance to learn the violin and I enjoyed being a member of its orchestra. I met Matt and his brother, John, after grade 8. Matt lived just down the street from me on Courtland Ave. We used to play baseball at Victoria Park. We called our team, The Vigilantes, Matt's suggestion. He was a great guy!

June 19: Bernard Katz: Dear Matt - So good to have known you even for the short time we became friends, after meeting at Sunnybrook Hospital in TO for a coffee during the difficult days when your brother was there in a coma. You are already missed, but memories of you stay on. To echo the 'bard': "May flights of angels sing thee to thy rest".

Deborah Thomas: The Board of the Ex Libris-Association, where Matt was active for some years, sends their condolences on the loss of their friend and colleague and your husband, father, and friend. His wonderful sense of humour, which reminded us often not to take ourselves too seriously, will be much missed. While we respect his wish to end his life on his own terms, his absence among us will be deeply felt. The news of his passing has been shared with the Ex Libris-membership.

June 20: Miriam & Carsten Schernekau: We will treasure our time together especially during the lockdown. You were a true friend providing Carsten with lots of reading material. Thank you from the bottom of our hearts. Miriam & Carsten

Evelyn Reid: I was privileged to know Matt as a friend for almost 50 years. During that time, I witnessed his kindness, generosity, compassion, and humour. Matt was a good man. We often recommended books to each other; my reading was enhanced by his recommendations. I offer this quote which, when I read it the first time, left me in tears as Matt's absence does today: "Sometimes the people you love leave you even when they don't want to, and you shatter into pieces. You may not be able to find all those pieces again because when they left, they took a few with them. It hurts, but the pain eventually becomes bearable and even sacred because it's how you carry the people you've lost with you. And if you're lucky you can one day see that the hollow spots you carry are in the shape of their face or their hands or the love, they gave you. Those holes ache, but they are the monument to the lost, a travelling sacred place to honour them and remind you of how to love enough to leave your own marks on others."
Jenny Lawson, Broken (in the best possible way) 2021/2022

*****

Afterthought about Matt: When I tore my shoulder tendons, it took a year to get to a pain management clinic in Hamilton, an hour's drive from Vineland. I wonder if the system were better, that Matt could have gotten to a pain management regimen, and also had things improved for his feeding tube, if he would still be alive. I had an idealistic image of him managing his pain, and finding ways to exercise and keep moving, even with a walker. Maybe, taking a painting course at a local college to produce lovely watercolors or a creative writing course?

I know that Joni Eareckson Tada lived a productive life after a diving accident at the age of 17 which made her a quadriplegic. She's lived 55 years in a wheelchair. She is 71 years old and lives in Baltimore, Maryland.

During her two-year rehabilitation, when she was young, she experienced anger, depression, suicidal thoughts, and religious doubts. Had MAiD ended her life then, many people would have been deprived of her artwork and her inspirational books. She learned to paint with a brush between her teeth. She also wrote books with voice recognition hardware. Life does not have to end if you find another way of living. But it helps if one has a timely medical system and a good pain management program.

Matt went the way he did. There was little choice. Canada was Canada with a failing system in 2023.

15
Rose Finlay

My wife and I sat at our TV trays eating lunch when I noted a "news ticker" flash by in the bottom of the screen. This was after Matt had published his own news on Caring Bridge that he chose MAiD. In fact, Matt had already waved goodbye to the crowd below at the pergola of his Oxford Estates apartment building and had already been cremated.

I told my wife that if I were cornered in the failed health care system with chronic pain, I'd want to go like Matt with the help of MAiD with an immediate cremation to follow. I figure funeral homes are making enough money as it is with traditional burials.

So, the "news ticker" at the bottom of the TV screen said that a single mother of 3 children in Bowmanville, Ontario, a quadriplegic who was restricted to her wheelchair was applying for MAiD. She observed that it was easier to access MAiD than ODSP, the Ontario Disability Support Program. MAiD could be approved within a 2-month period, whereas ODSP required an 8 month, or more, wait time.

Her dilemma was clear. The system had failed her.

*Source: **CBC News, article by Tyler Cheese, posted June 22, 2023**

Rose Finlay, 33, had been restricted to her wheelchair since she was 17, becoming a quadriplegic since a diving accident. The cause of her accident and her age are similar to what happened to Joni Eareckson Tada.

"I've been very ill," Finlay said. "I've been bedridden for the last year, so my quality of life has significantly decreased."

As a single, handicapped mother it has not been easy to support her family of 3 boys. She'd supported her family from disability advocacy work through her company, "Inclusive Solutions". Money from that also paid for her own support workers. She was able to live reasonably.

However, about a year ago, her care workers moved on to other jobs. That's when her health deteriorated. She applied to the Ontario Disability Support Program where she was told over the phone, that the wait time was at least six to eight months long.

While spinning in circles with the red tape, Rose Finlay got recurring infections which threatened to turn into sepsis. Finlay applied for MAiD last March.

Ron Anicin, spokesman for ODSP, told CBC Toronto that applications for assistance has been growing, where patients have even considered MAiD "because they feel like they're running out of options." Nothing is clear about how long a patient looking for ODSP help needs to wait.

"That's a big problem," he said. "If people are even considering going for MAiD because of poor social assistance rates, then that is something that definitely needs to be looked at, that needs to be fixed, that needs to be repaired."

I chuckled when I read this last comment by Ron Anicin. It was so political, so correct. One often hears the phraseology of "we must investigate this," "we must have a study on it," when nothing ever is really done! But who can blame Mr. Anicin when the system is so broken that nothing, he can do personally, can fix it.

Rose Finlay has a right to feel frustrated. "That tells me that our government is not prioritizing the lives of disabled people and that it is easier to let disabled people go than it is to actually give them the assistance that they need."

Finlay is cornered into applying for MAiD with her recurring infections. "It's not what I want," she said. "But if I don't receive the support that I need, the outcome is the same. If I get to a point where I am really sick and basically terminally ill anyways, I would like to have other options."

What happens to Finlay's three boys if she gives up her life with MAiD? How much will the state have to pay to put her boys into the foster care system. What a dilemma!

Rose Finlay's dilemma is an example of how the parameters for MAiD have changed and broadened to threaten the lives of people in wheelchairs.

*****

I watched a movie through *YouTube* recently, entitled "The Humanity Bureau," starring Nicolas Cage. With global warming, parts of the American Midwest are turned into a desert in the near future. The Humanity Bureau, a government agency, takes over to manage this economic recession. Members of society are ranked on a "productivity quotient." If unproductive, they are exiled to a colony known as "New Eden." Little do people know that New Eden is an extermination camp. Nicolas Cage, as Noah Kross, hates this aspect of his job of ranking people because he finds out that unproductive people are exterminated.

Thank goodness for social watchdogs, especially writers, who research and disseminate the truth and question political decisions. Let's hope our legal system and the Supreme Court is up to the task, as well, to guard the vulnerable.

One can understand a sick person's urge to get away from his or her pain, but if eligibility becomes too broad, then removing a life would not only be immoral but criminal, as well. Who knows where the line would jump to, from irredeemably ill people to non-productive members of society?

I can understand the need for MAiD in excruciating circumstances but am cautious when eligibility for it broadens to people who are not deemed to face an imminent and near future death where, if they got timely care, they could still lead productive lives.

I like what CARP, the advocacy group for seniors, is suggesting, i.e., staying in your home longer where you can age with dignity. If you were funded for home care, such care is less expensive, according to CARP, than going into a seniors' home or to the hospital. Too many Canadians who require care at home, spend too long on wait lists for the support and quality of life they really need. Does our Premier Ford in Ontario ever listen to classical radio where CARP advertises their excellent suggestion for funding home care?

Quality of life involves a flexible definition, and the law must intervene, of course, to advocate for the mentally ill and those who could still function, if services were available. We must not approach a future society where, as in the movie, "Soylent Green," a person is euthanized when he simply gets tired of life and says, "I've had enough." People end up on a conveyor belt and are processed into protein tablets in an overpopulated, starving New York. Writers, artists, and film makers, I think, are our watchdogs to make sure that scary futuristic worlds do not become reality.

   Let's hope our politicians and our Supreme Court Justices are also our watchdogs with a conscience for a "just society". I'm old enough to remember Pierre Elliott Trudeau working for a vision of "Canada to be a just society" way back in September of 1968.

16
My Friend, Adam

I've got two friends now who used Medical Assistance in Dying. Matt Scholtz and Adam.

I did not use Adam's full name out of respect for his parents. They shied away from publicity. They also did not use Caring Bridge and preferred to connect to close friends only by e-mail.

I knew Adam used MAiD only from private e-mails and visits to his parents at the seniors' home. Adam was celiac. He had terrible food allergies and suffered from 5 ulcers in his stomach. He subsisted on special shakes, occasionally bits of chicken, fish, and rice. He was sick all the time, couldn't eat right and couldn't sleep right. When he lived in Toronto, he was under the care of a psychiatrist for persistent depressive disorders. No wonder!

I don't have a detailed story on Adam. As I said, there was no blog like Caring Bridge, plus his parents were reticent about their family problems. Who wants to listen to other people's problems anyway? Human nature!

Adam died just 10 days after his 49th birthday. He stood maybe 5'6" tall. He was skinny as a rail and must have weighed a smidge under 100 pounds. He was a delicate fellow with a delicate soul. He was a gifted person, a guitar player, a writer, a singer, and composer of lovely songs.

Adam came from talented Jewish parents. They moved a few houses down from us some years ago. I found it ironic that their house faced our Mennonite church, whereas they were Jewish by birth and were confirmed Atheists.

The mother was a renowned Shakespearean scholar and a writer of books about the holocaust and black history. The father was a skilled composer of classical music.

They were both Oxfordians, something I had never heard of, showing my lack of education in certain areas. Of course, when I was going through school, I never liked Shakespeare anyway.

An Oxfordian is a scholar who says that Shakespeare did not write his plays! The real bard was the Earl of Oxford who simply gave credit to Shakespeare because it was unseemly for nobility to write plays during the 16th and 17th centuries.

Adam was, of course, quite learned coming from such educated parents. Adam, with parents like that, was a skilled "wordsmith" in his own right. I'm sure he never reached his full potential because of his ailments.

Adam had medical and financial support when he lived in Toronto but that all stopped when he moved in with his parents here in Vineland out of Toronto's jurisdiction and support network.

I loved visiting the family because we'd talk about art, music, and books. Actually, these people were responsible for the fire lit in me to write my first murder mystery, about an honor killing at Ball's Falls. The father was my proofreader. The book was The New Crusades and subsequently, The New Crusades: The Sequel.

Adam's mother was falling and forgetting things while living in Vineland opposite our church. She eventually had to be put in a home. The father sold the house in Vineland and he and Adam moved in together into a little house in St. Catharine's.

Adam's allergies got worse. He asked his dad to help him commit suicide one day. Of course, when the dad could not bring himself to do this, Adam jumped off a bridge in St. Catharine's. He was rescued when someone saw his body below the bridge. He survived with broken bones. His attempted suicide only made things worse since hospitals were closing wards at this time during the Pandemic because of Covid. The whole system seemed to have come to a stop. Their excuse? They had to keep a number of beds open, in case there was a rush of Covid patients. How stupid was that?

Adam got no help from any psychiatric doctor in Niagara, nor help for his food allergies. There was no referral to a pain clinic to manage his worsening chronic pain.

Waiting times were crazy. Someone coming into the emergency ward at the St. Catharine's hospital would have to wait 5 hours, at least, to be seen. This was ironic in that Adam gave his free time to help society, volunteering to help the homeless and also man the Food Bank. When he needed help himself, there was none there.

Adam was sent home, after his attempted suicide, and the application for MAiD was filled out. Within 10 days, poor Adam was dead. There was no celebration of life, none that I was invited to and no website like Caring Bridge. The obituary said he passed away "under the caring and compassionate supervision of MAiD professionals."

*****

I wrote a book, most of the story imagined, about a man named Adam who suffered from depression,

allergies, and a failed medical system. The book was called
<u>Joshua's Journey</u>.

I wish that I could have had a talent for music and
singing like Adam. Despite his ailments, he wrote and sang
lovely lyrics with a soft voice producing a collection of his
songs in a CD entitled, "Little Car". He imagined himself
driving off with his guitar to become famous in LA. How
idealistic!

> Most of my body
> Don't work well,
> Health ain't a word
> It can spell.
> Most of my body
> Don't work well,
> But my heart is doing fine,
> 'Cause once again you're mine.

17
Dear Adam

After Adam's attempted suicide and unsuccessful bid for help in the hospital, he recovered enough to move back into his father's house. My wife and I hadn't heard from them for many months. That must have been a stressful time for both of them, living in such close quarters in that little house.

Then on a Sunday evening, we got a phone call from Adam's dad that Adam was scheduled to die in three days, on a Wednesday morning, with doctor assisted suicide. We were told not to tell anyone, for the time being, but we were welcome to send Adam an e-mail which the father would read to him. We composed two heart-felt messages:

Monday, June 21, 2021
Dear Adam:

We are writing you this letter with real sadness in our hearts. We had hoped and prayed that the doctors would find a way to alleviate your pain, but we understand that that could not be done. We support you in the decision you have made to find a way to end the pain. We cannot understand what you have lived through these past years, but we do know what it is like to live with daily pain and how that affects every aspect of your life. Now, our prayer for you and your family is peace and comfort.

Adam, we will always remember you as a quiet and gentle man with great talents and great compassion. The CD of your songs made us smile, laugh, and cry. Every time we listen to it in the future, we will think fondly of you. Marjorie loves looking at the picture of you on the back cover where you are smiling in happier times. She also remembers each time she ran into you at the Superstore, shopping with your dad. Even though you were not feeling well, you always asked how John was doing. As we said, you are a man of great talents and great compassion. We feel privileged to have gotten to know you.

We will continue to befriend and support your parents in any way we can. If we could be there with you right now, we would want to give you a great big hug. We care.

Your friends

_____

Tuesday, June 22, 2021
Dear Adam:

I think we inherited the two rabbits from your dad's old backyard on Menno Street. Some evenings, I just sit on our lawn-chair on the back deck and watch the furry critters scurry around foraging. They look well fed.

My wife's Opa in the old days would sit on his porch and take pot shots at rabbits with his .22. Since it was in suburbia, Aunt Irene confiscated the rifle and hid it.

It's a cool evening. I went for a bicycle ride to the local school and back. Adam, I remember when you would walk around a couple of blocks here in Vineland. It was always nice seeing you do your "401".

Had health blessed you, I could have become closer friends with you. I was really impressed with your songs in that CD. I even had the notion that you might teach me to play the guitar someday. As it is, I am just glad that I got to know you and appreciate your dry wit. Not everybody around here catches cute references to authors like Kafka or composers like Debussy. Your whole family has been a civilizing experience for me.

My wife and I are so glad that we have your CD. If I had a wish for you, I'd wish that you were healthy and that you had a job as a DJ at some talk show on a radio station in Toronto. You take personal experiences and expand those moments into actual songs. You are a man with great imagination and with very poetic feelings.

I miss being silly and smart-alecky with you because I know you can take me with a grain of salt, maybe a whole shaker. Even with your talent to come back with clever quips, when I joke with you, I know you also see the profound things in life. The universe will be less without you.

My wife and I just love that photo of you and the golden retriever on the back of your CD cover. We wish you well on the journey you must take on Wednesday. May all your pain be left far behind!

Your caring friends

_____

A note here:
I've left last names out in this story to respect Adam's parents' wish for privacy. My wife also does not like her name used in my writings and hates the internet.

As a Christian, I had some ethical questions about Adam's choice to exit life. Was this a right thing to do in Canada's medical system? I could understand it, however, the crying need to end pain, God, or no God.

This way to end life for a human being has become permissible now in a humane system of care.

If God does not exist, then my ethical questions are irrelevant. But since I am a believer, I find this specific question irritatingly relevant: "Where do good Atheists Go When They Die?" Because Adam was an Atheist and a good guy!

I hate to think that oblivion is the final fate for all of us, no matter whether we are good, indifferent, or outrageously bad in this life. But if God does exist, I want to feel that my friend Adam gets a fair deal in eternity.

18
Vineland Friendships

I first got to know Adam's mother and father when they moved from Toronto into our little community in Vineland only a few houses down from us. They were Jewish and they were Atheists. We rarely spoke about religion, but they knew both the Old and New Testaments better than I did.

It was Adam's mother who prompted my journey into writing and publishing my own books. Like I said, Adam's mother was a novelist and Shakespearean scholar. The father was a respected classical music composer. They knew Kerry Stratton, the famous Torontonian conductor personally, when they lived in the big city. In fact, I knew Kerry too. He was my conductor in the Grande Prairie Symphony Orchestra when I was a young man.

Anyway, having such educated people down the street lit a fire in me to start writing. At the time when I wrote my first novel, The New Crusades, ISIS was making news. I debated about using a pseudonym to protect my anonymity because religious extremists can be crazy. Look at what happened to Salman Rushdie! At the time, honor killing seemed to happen regularly in Canada. My story was a fiction based on an honor killing at Ball's Falls. The brother fled to Syria after killing his sister. Adam's father agreed to proofread my first literary effort.

I was amused when the family first moved into our community. At the time, they were the only ones who put up Christmas lights on a little tree in their front lawn. The wife liked the pretty colours. We not only had literature in common but at the time, I also played violin in the Peninsula Orchestra, so we enjoyed classical music together.

My wife and I were invited over during the Christmas Season to light the Menorah candle during Hanukkah. Adam's family still celebrated Jewish traditions, though they were confirmed Atheists. They did not spurn other people's beliefs.

They enjoyed a good talk about the nature of the universe, about evolution, creation and even the concept of God, which when it got to an impasse or a sensitive area, was left alone. We'd settle for a replay of a Star Trek episode on TV.

At times, we did have meaningful talks about our different religions. They, speaking about the respect they had for Jewish traditions, though they did not believe, and me, talking about my need for a Faith as a Christian. I liked Saint Peter's advice regarding the exchange of ideas and imparting one's opinion about one's own Faith in a civil manner:

> 1 Peter 3:15, NIV: "But in your hearts revere Christ as Lord. Always be prepared to give an answer to everyone who asks you to give the reason for the hope that you have. But do this with gentleness and respect."

I just wish that I were more versed in Scripture and that I could speak more intelligently about my Faith...but I've never had a good memory. I've never been convinced of God's existence, either by logic or intelligence, but by my weakness and need to believe in a Supreme Being.

*****

Adam moved to our little village into his parents' home when he found it difficult to make ends meet in Toronto. Adam gave me the CD he made of his songs which he composed and in which he played guitar and sang beautifully with his rich baritone voice.

Adam was a chip off the old block from his dad and mom, inheriting a knack for poetry and music. He had a dry sense of humour. He knew a lot about philosophy and religion, though like his folks, he had no use for religion.

When Adam's mother lost her balance several years ago, the father sold the house across from the church and bought a tiny fixer upper in the city. The mother ended up in a seniors' home where more care could be provided because of her poor balance and failing health. Adam got a concession from the administration to bring a roll-up bed into his mother's room, so he could occasionally sleep there, keep her company, and help her with her panic attacks.

At other times, Adam and his father lived together in their little house, coping the best they could with their changed circumstances.

It was during this time that Adam's health also declined. The huge wait times did not help with his ulcers, his allergies and with his life. The Pandemic, of course, made things intolerable!

19
The Question of God

All my dreams
Pass before my eyes, a curiosity.

Song by Kansas-1978

As I said, if God does not exist, this whole concern about an afterlife, where an Atheist goes and in fact, where we all go, is like dust in the wind, blown away, worth nothing.

But mankind has always had hopes of something better and beyond himself which has sustained people's struggles and sufferings throughout the ages.

Unfortunately, my idea of God and your idea of God have not always agreed, and people have cut each other's throats to prove they are right. Mark Twain, in his inimical cynicism had a lot to say about religion where he jokingly said he did an experiment by putting men of different religions in a cage, to see how they got along. When he came back, there wasn't a specimen left alive. They took their theological differences to a higher court.

That kind of earthly disagreement is the reason for "Holy Wars". What an antithetical concept to have a "Holy" War, where priests bless combatants before they go out to kill each other! How can a war be Holy? The concept is an oxymoron which caused the deaths of thousands on the basis of a difference in beliefs. Organized religion can be so destructive in the name of God who is supposed to be all-merciful and good.

Introspective people have always looked at Holy Wars as stupid. It's an old story often revisited. In our specific case, we don't need to rehash such a large problem in the history of mankind because we have something more specific in mind. The question of "Where do good Atheists go in the afterlife?"

I am not convinced by Thomas Aquinas' approach through his "Quinque Viae" that God exists, which are his five proofs for God. Yet, he made a good effort.

Let's assume that God does indeed exist, otherwise I would have nothing to write about here. Richard Dawkins is probably smirking at this point, but what the heck. This is not a full-proof treatise out to prove anything. Like the many people in history behind me who have pondered eternal questions, this is just a simple inquiry.

The scientific method is supposed to make the God of the Gaps smaller and smaller as more things get explained. However, even if all these Gaps were explained away, I find that human nature would still seek for help from something beyond.

I call this the God of the Needs. That is a basis for Faith and a support for trials, suffering and even dying. I do not care about Dawkins' intellectual suicide. I admit my weakness and my need for spiritual comfort.

I was actually comforted by Adam's obituary which read:

> On Wednesday, June 23, 2021, ten days after his 49th birthday, Adam passed away peacefully under the caring and compassionate supervision of the MAiD (Medical Assistance in Dying) professionals. We are very grateful to them as they also helped see us through such a difficult time. Adam was a kind and generous man who cared more about other people's

well-being than his own. He volunteered at the Food Bank and helped the homeless and unemployed cut through bureaucracies to get the assistance they needed... In lieu of flowers or food, please consider a donation to the MAiD House in Toronto.

20
Kenneth Wayne Janzen

The gravestone reads, "Loving Husband, Father, and Son. Kenneth "Ken" Wayne Janzen August 5, 1970 – January 18, 2008. The bottom of the stone has a strip of piano keys which symbolizes Ken's gift in music.

I used a photo of that gravestone for the book cover of one of my murder mysteries, erasing Ken's name through Photoshop and inserting the title, <u>Things Have Gotta Get Better Than This!</u> I thought this was clever. Kenny would not mind and might even like the sardonic irony of the title.

I want to thank Scott Brettell, a dear friend of Ken's, who was adept in computers, for saving Ken's original Blog, so that I could get a copy and write a trilogy on my former dear brother-in-law. The trilogy's title was <u>Time in a Bottle</u>.

Like Adam, my former brother-in-law, was multi-gifted, a singer, a painter, a composer, and keyboard player. He was also a web designer, earning awards for the best websites in the Niagara Peninsula. I asked him to make me a website, but he was so busy earning a living that he had no time. I enrolled in night school at Mohawk College and eventually designed my own site through persistence and hard work.

As I sit in my study and write this book, I look up to the left wall and see two framed photos. One photo is of Kenny and me making silly peace signs behind our heads. The other is my Webmaster's Diploma from Mohawk

College which I earned from my night school credits in 2007.

Anyway, Kenny was the family computer guru. If we had trouble, he would come over with his Timmy's coffee in hand and fix our computers.

Except for Kenny's special genius in the digital world, he reminded me so much of Adam. Kenny had a 4-octave range and could sing harmony to himself from tenor to bass, composing his own melodies and lyrics. Kenny came from a Mennonite musical family, where singing in the church choir was a regular family thing. Kenny expanded his musical gifts into keyboard playing, then manipulating the synthesizer via the computer. He even made a CD of his own songs, "My Sentiments Exactly". We also have a painting of his on our great room wall.

Kenny fought fiercely for his life. He had two wonderful children, Braeden 2, and Darriane 6 back in 2007. A pretty wife and a thriving web design business. He had lots to live for. He died at the age of 37, after such a long battle, a fight we all followed through "Ken's Health and Wellness Blog". How could a fair God, we asked, do this to someone so young?

In 2007, he went to the family doctor with a sniffle and cough. There was a suspicious blotch on the x-ray, and we found out he had lung cancer. The next 9 months were horrendous. Kenny launched his Health and Wellness Blog, similar to Caring Bridge. I tracked his story and had lots to write about in his battle with lung cancer.

At the time, however, there was no medical assistance in dying, so MAiD was not available to him. He had to ride his lung cancer out by himself right to the very end. I asked my wife, if MAiD had existed back then, would Kenny have chosen this way out. My wife said, No. He was determined to fight for life. But I'm not so sure, because he was in terrible pain and the whole 9 months was a slow slide downhill. When he died, he looked like something out of a concentration camp and his 6-foot frame must have weighed all of 100 pounds, maybe less. There was so much hope and so much support from friends and relatives in his blog.

*****

As I tracked his postings through the blog and people's responses, I came up with enough material to write a Trilogy on Kenny's suffering. The title of the trilogy, as I said, was <u>Time in a Bottle</u>.

If I could save time in a bottle
The first thing that I'd like to do
Is to save every day 'til eternity passes away
Just to spend them with you.
Jim Croce 1973

21
Ken's Health
And Wellness Blog

MARCH 2007

CT scans and Surgeons - Oh My!
31. March 2007 @ 07:45
Well, another update. I also now have a confirmed appointment with a Thoracic surgeon for Tuesday, April 10 at 12:30pm. I was hoping to get in sooner - like on Friday the 6th just after my CT scan - but apparently no self-respecting doctor seems to work Good Friday or Easter Monday. Oh Well....
The Medical Mystery that is Me :) | Comments (0)

The Saga Continues
29. March 2007 @ 10:50
As of today, I now have a confirmed CAT Scan appointment, at the St. Catharine's General, on Tuesday, April 3rd, at 4:30pm.

Hopefully I will be able to see the Thoracic Surgeon shortly thereafter to discuss the CAT Scan results and go over how the subsequent biopsy will work.

The Medical Mystery that is Me :) | Comments (7)

APRIL 2007

And I Rage!
27. April 2007 @ 14:21
Today is another one of those very bad days.

I have been given my official prognosis by my oncologist and with much sorrow I will share it with you now. If I had no conventional treatment (chemo) they give me 6 months to live. With chemo that number jumps to a *whopping* 12-18 months.

So, I sit here typing and I RAGE!!! In between the bouts of tears, I RAGE! I clench my fists till I can clench no more – I shake those fists at the heavens and shout to the Lord; "Why?!", "Why Me?!" "Why should my beautiful 5-year-old daughter and wonderful 20-month-old son have to grow up without me as their father?!", "Why should I have to be the one to have to leave my beautiful wife, my soulmate and best friend?", "Why am I the one who has to leave all my friends behind?", "Was I not good enough? Living enough, caring enough?" ....and I RAGE!!! I rage until I cannot handle the wracking pain of my sobs anymore.

And I suppose this is a natural reaction, as I am only human and trying to seek answers where there are no obvious answers to be had. All I can do now is trust that God does have a plan for me and my family.

Please forgive me! I have not given up. Not by a long shot! It's just that coming to terms with your own mortality in light of a really poor prognosis can make even the most positive (and humorous) of us crack under pressure.

Change of Focus
28. April 2007 @ 10:23

If you look - just over there...you will see it with me! The light of hope at the end of the tunnel! That light, which I now see, is wholly representative and made up of all the love, words, prayers, and thoughts you all gave to us yesterday. So brightly it shines!!

That light is responsible for pulling me out of yesterday's quagmire. At first in the day, I couldn't see it - it was a very dark day. Then as the day grew on into the night, the light grew so bright and powerful, you could not avoid seeing it - it was everywhere! Enveloping me and my family with a blanket of comfort and peace. As I have said to you, countless times already, thank-you is not enough and yet I don't have the words to adequately express how I feel, I wish I did! I wish I could express even the tiniest portion of the love and gratitude I feel - but I don't know how...

If it was last year, I would have written a song for you all. Written it specifically for each and every one of you! But as most of you know, God has seen fit to allow me to have laryngitis - so even that avenue of release and escape which I loved is not available to me.

All I can do now is write here in this blog, so that means that this blog and my communication with all of you is my new escape -
So... focusing on this blog combined with my fierce determination to beat this bodily invader is my change of focus!!

Will I still rage? Of course. Will I still cry? You betcha. However, I will channel all my rage against this cancer. I will channel all your love, prayers, and tears to my heart - as   they   heal   me   each   and   every   day!

Do I know what tomorrow brings? well, no. But you know what?
With God, my family and all of you by my side I don't care!! BRING IT ON BABY!! I know that everything will be alright.

I love you all! Ken
The Medical Mystery that is Me :) | Comments (836)

Comments
Re: Change of Focus by Marilyn & Jerry
28. April 2007 @ 10:57

And We Love You
Too!!

[Marilyn and Jerry are Kenny's sister and brother-in-law.]
A poem was forwarded from Helen Steiner Rice:

> Often we pause and wonder
> When we kneel down to pray---
> Can God really hear
> The prayers that we say....
> But if we keep praying
> And talking to HIM
> He'll brighten the soul
> that was clouded and dim
> And as we continue
> Our burden seems lighter,
> Our sorrow is softened
> And our outlook is brighter---

For though we feel helpless
And alone when we start,
Our prayer is the key
That opens the heart,
And as our heart opens
The dear Lord comes in
And the prayer that we felt
We could never begin
Is so easy to say
For the Lord understands
And gives us new strength
By the touch of HIS Hands.
Amen

When your storm started tossing you around it felt like I was holding on to the boat but not able to get in to help you. I started reading a poem book called Heart Gifts by Helen Steiner Rice. A dear friend Jane Martens gave it to me in 1989. Many of these poems have calmed my inner storms over the past years. We can't get in your boat with you, but we will hang on to help calm it. When the storm hits again do not fear, we are hanging on, riding it out with you.
Again
We love you and are praying for you with every breath we take.

Marilyn.

22
Huh? What class?

UPDATE to the "Possibilities" Post Below!!!
15. May 2007 @ 18:28
Well, I just received a call at 5:30pm today from the medical oncologist I saw yesterday in Toronto. You can basically forget that entire "Possibilities" post below as she now thinks that I'm back to being classified as stage four.

Apparently yesterday she did not have my "operative report" (from my biopsy surgery) and she did not see my most recent CT scan written report (it was faxed to Princess Margaret Hospital in the early afternoon) - whereas the radiation oncologist did see it.

Anyway, the medical oncologist is now saying that upon her review of these reports - she now thinks I am in stage 4 - which again I think is a load of CRAP! They were all set to do more tests including a new CT scan and more, but those have now been **canceled**. HORSES#@T!!! Now, I could accept this diagnosis if this Toronto doctor had done any further tests - but she did NOT! So, I am now completely at the mercy of our laughable Canadian medical system and can get no help! My only choice now is to raise some funds and head south of the border. I feel somewhat like Mel Gibson in the movie "Conspiracy

Theory"...except for one difference - I have God and all of you on my side!

And by the way, just like here in Niagara, this new medical oncologist did NOT do a biopsy of my lower lymph nodes or ANY other tests for that matter - yet it is because of those very nodes that she has revised and reversed her diagnosis from yesterday. I understand that she is VERY experienced in cancer diagnosis and all - but if it was you or your child, wouldn't you want to know for SURE! Wouldn't you perform any and every available test? Why can I not still go for the Brain MRI and the CT scan? Why have these options been taken away from me?

I mean, 2 of the lymph nodes in question actually SHRANK from one CT scan to another - how in the name of all things holy does a node SHRINKING become a cancer indicator? Oh well, I'm not a doctor, I'm just the patient - what the heck do I know?!

So, I ask...what gives with all these cancer doctors just ASSUMING??!! These are supposed to be THE top cancer professionals in our country - whom I thought, as of yesterday, had at least SOME professional curiosity and would actually try to get to the bottom of things! But alas, that is not the case AGAIN!

You know what this is like? It's like a mechanic reading some reports from another mechanic about your car that just isn't working right. Your mechanic reads those OLD and fairly limited third-party reports and then looks at some older and newer photos of your car and out of the blue...comes up with a diagnosis that your shocks are gone.   HOW   DO   THEY   KNOW??!!

Don't fear though - I have not given up hope!!! I'm just REALLY   angry   right   now...

The fact that I have fewer spots on my lung and that my nodes are shrinking are small miracles - let's just keep the faith that there are larger miracles to come! I have MUCH more faith in God than I do in our medical system. He is the ultimate healer!

Funny thing too - we literally JUST got an email from the other doctor in Cleveland. he didn't want to say what 'stage' I was in without further testing...hmmm.... imagine that! So, guess what he is recommending for further tests? A PET Scan and an MRI of the brain...sound familiar?? I'm going to call him within the next few days (he gave us his number) to see if those procedures can be done down there in the USA and also to see how much they would cost -
seeing as I can no longer have them done here in Canada.

*****

Thanks again to all of you for your words of encouragement. In my darkest hours I read through this blog again and again and gain strength from your words. In your words I find joy. In your words I find hope!

In God's word, I find all that and now...peace!

OK – I'm done venting now – sorry 'bout that!
I'll be posting again in the morning, so stay tuned.

The Medical Mystery that is Me :) | Comments (13)

23
Back to Values

The Demise of Dinner
20. May 2007 @ 12:16

You know it's funny. Here I am, Ken the "cancer boy" writing daily entries on this blog and more often than not I'm 'preaching' about the value of time - how precious it is and the fact that we should all take the time to slow down and smell the roses –
when apparently, I'm having a hard time practicing what I 'preach'.

We have been so busy the past few weeks – understandably? Well, I guess so. But still we've been running around like "chickens-with-our-heads-cut-off" (to use that horrible analogy). Appointments here, tests there, naps squeezed in here and there, treatments over yonder and so on. Just keep this all in mind as I ramble for a second...

Sue and I were sitting in our kitchen on the evening of May the 18th (yes, the 15 year anniversary of the night we met) and we were lucky enough to have Shirley (MAW!) come over and baby sit for us for just a few hours so we could go out and be a couple - instead of being "Momma and Daddy". For those of you that have had the privilege of meeting both Sue and her mom, seeing them both in action you soon come to realize where Sue gets her spunk, her zest for life and her undying love and devotion. I can wholeheartedly say — it runs in the family!

So, apparently, does the ability for BOTH of them to sense when I am doing something wrong or stupid from over a kilometer away...and then comes the follow up ability of being able to throw a phone book at me with such accuracy as to startle an army sharpshooter! OUCH!!!...Ok just kidding about the phone book thing. ☺

Anyway, over the last 15 years, Shirley has truly become another mom - or MAW! as I love to call her — to me and I have come to love and respect her more than she will ever know. Ohhh...and by the way, she just LOVES it when I call her...MAW!! She says it sounds like a dying crow. Anything I can do to get under her skin for fun! After all, that IS the job of a son-in-law, isn't it?? .... haha!

OK...OK...back to the story. We were sitting in the kitchen chatting with MAW! when she observed that I was eating a very late supper while all the rest of the family had eaten already. She asked me why and I made my excuses, but it wasn't good enough for MAW! She launched into a mini-rant about how families just don't spend time together anymore — specifically at dinnertime — and how it's affecting our social fabric, etc... etc...
And you know what? She's SO right!

Here I am, 'preaching' in my blog about cherishing every moment and I'm missing something as crucial (and as simple) as dinner with my family. Shirley's comments then led me to ask myself...what ever happened to our family dinner?

When I was young, we ALWAYS had dinner at the table as a family – it was just a given. And for the most part so did everyone else we knew. Nowadays though, with everyone's hectic lifestyle – it seems like we all just grab what we can when we can. And we wonder why we have lost the ability to communicate with our spouse or our kids…. Why? Because we don't take the time to talk to them! We truly are ships passing in the night with the only light breaking through the darkness, coming from a cellphone.

It seems like such a simple little silly thing – but I truly think the demise of dinner IS having a negative influence on our family circles as a whole. So, what can we do? Well, as hard as it is to balance our schedules – maybe we can try to make time to sit down together as a family and just talk. Not sit in front of the TV as a family – but sit at the table. At first – there may be awkward silences and stares….

but I'm sure things will get better, and the communication will start!

To those of you who still practice the 'art' of dinner as a family I stand and applaud you! For those of you who don't, and if the 'non-family-dinner' scenario sounds familiar in your house, I need to ask you...
will you work to change it? I know I will!

When this whole realization hit me, I felt like an idiot. I WANT to spend more time with my kids, and I was missing out on such a simple way to do it! Jeez, talk about an "OOPS!"

Anyway, thanks MAW! For your insight and wisdom! Hopefully because of you we will all work together to stop the demise of dinner.

Till tomorrow.

PS – I hope all my fellow Canadians are having a wonderful long weekend! Enjoy!

The Medical Mystery that is Me :) | Comments (144)

24
I'm What??!!
Again??!!

24 May 2007 @11:53

Well, before I get to today...I should fill you all in on what happened yesterday. Around 1:30pm we got a call from our family doctor who told us that he had just gotten a "written" report in from Princess Margaret Hospital and he would like to see us about it right away. *Ok*, I thought. *This can be good news or bad news.* And then my mind continued to race; *They didn't do any more tests when we were up there except for bloodwork and an x-ray...so what is this all about??!* With a further shrug of my shoulders, Sue and I piled into the car and drove down to the doctors. On the way over Suzie looked at me and softly asked "are you scared?" "Of course, I am" I replied, "who wouldn't be." We reached out and grabbed each other's hands. And yet again my mind churned as I thought *what's the worst that could happen...to the docs I'm already a dead man walking anyway* So I left it at that and resigned myself that since I could not control what was on this 'report' I would not worry about it anymore. I enjoyed my wife's company and the music on the radio for the rest of the trip.

So we get in there and get to see the doctor after only a 3–4-minute wait (He's usually pretty good that way). So, he strolls in and throws a report down on the desk that is indeed from Princess Margaret Hospital. He has a 'scrunched up' kinda perturbed look on his face and again I start to worry. But he starts to read...."upon further review of his files, we think Mr. Janzen actually may be in **stage 3** of his cancer and therefore eligible for radiation, surgery and   other   curative   approaches...."

WHAT!!!??   ...   **WHAT!!??**

We just heard this garbage last Monday (the 14th) from these clowns. And then they kyboshed the whole thing by phone the next day telling me that OOPS! upon even FURTHER review I indeed was stage 4. So NOW - a week and a half later... my doctor gets a report dated May the 23rd that says I'm in stage 3 and that my case will be presented to the "tumor board' at the hospital on May 25th.

All of us just sat there and shook our heads and wondered aloud if these "lauded" and "celebrated" doctors up there in Toronto actually can tell their ass from a hole in the ground! My family doctor said it best; "This just isn't right!" he said, "They are flip-flopping you around here...what kind of people are they anyway".

Well, after a few more minutes of discussion, we came to the conclusion that - even though the report was dated today and referenced the tumour board on the 25th - the report HAS to be some kind of mistake. So, we jumped in the van and rushed over to Sue's Mom's house - which is only about 5 min away from the doctors.
...   and   Sue   got   on   the   phone.

After about 5 min - she was able to get one of the interns familiar with my case on the phone who confirmed that yes - the report was just typed wrong. OOPS!!!! Their official diagnosis for me was still stage four lung cancer NOT stage three. I should sue these idiots for gross negligence and for causing mental anguish.

Anyway, I also found out from my doctor why they reversed their position last week (from stage 3 back to stage 4) OK, for those of you that don't remember - I'm considered stage 4 if my lower lymph nodes are cancerous (which we DON'T have a definitive answer for) and I'm considered stage 3 if they are not cancerous. The lower lymph nodes are the key. And remember - from the CT scan I had over a month ago to the one I had just recently, 2 of those nodes in question actually SHRANK!

So, last Monday or Tuesday sometime, before I got that infamous phone call... both the medical and radiation oncologists consulted with an infectious diseases specialist to determine if my Epstein-Barr (EB) could cause my lymph nodes to become enlarged.

It was the infectious disease doctors' rock-solid opinion that in NO way could my chronic Epstein-Barr cause my Lymph nodes to swell. <-- REMEMBER THIS!

So, this morning I did a quick Google search for "symptoms of Epstein-Barr virus" and TONS of pages came up. Here's an example.

Diagnose-me.com says and I quote:
> "...perhaps the most distinguishing mono (which is another name for Epstein Barr) symptom is enlarged

glands or lymph nodes, especially in the neck, but also in a person's armpit(s) and a person's groin."

And yet this infectious disease doctor KNOWS ALL! He says EB can't cause swelling of the lymph nodes so therefore it must be true. And the stupid thing is the other doctors just take it at face value without doing their 'homework'.
Jeez, just three minutes on the web and I was able to find out   TONS   of   info   on   this   topic.

One thing that I have well and truly learned is to ALWAYS remember people - the letters "Dr." in front of anybody's name does NOT make them God! Ask questions, LOTS of them and if your doctor doesn't want to answer you or find out answers for you - get another one! There are a few good docs left out there... and I am fortunate to call some of them very dear friends of mine. It's just unfortunate that they have no 'pull' in my particular case. Oh well.

But hey, who am I to doubt the docs? I'm just I'll ol' Ken! I'm not a doctor - what do I know. Well, a heck of a lot actually!

How much medical training have I had? Well, none.
But I do know my body and I do know that my father DID instill in me a drive to find answers and basic common sense - which I would venture to say that a lot of these high-and-mighty docs are seriously lacking.

OK I'll stop my little tirade on our healthcare system now!

25
"Bizarre Chapter in My Fight"

Kenny faced several frustrations during those early months of his battle against cancer in 2007. Dalton McGuinty was premier of Ontario. In 2014, when Kenny was already dead and buried, Kathleen Wynne took over that job. She promised all kinds of improvements to wait times in hospitals in the face of climbing hallway care...and of course, wait times. Nothing had changed, despite political promises.

In the meantime, during Kenny's struggle, the misdiagnosis, and the medical appointments within the "round and round we go" system, continued. Nobody was sure if Kenny was stage 4 or not. Technicians used terms like "almost definitely" A biopsy was recommended as 3 weeks already passed by in the medical communications circle. Kenny compared himself to a "pogo stick" hopping up and down in the system, not being grounded. He was also getting skinny like a pogo stick.

26 May 2007 @ 09:34
So begins the next bizarre chapter in my fight with the Canadian hospitals to get some definitive answers about the actual "stage" of my lung cancer.

Most of you all know what happened to us the other day...we got called in to our family doctors to go over a report that was just faxed to him from Toronto. Turns out that the report was an old one and it led to some serious confusion because of some typos in the dates in the body of the report (for the full story please read the post below entitled "I'm What??!! AGAIN??!!"

[Kenny listened to a third message on his answering machine.]

Third message
..."Hi this is Dr. [medical oncologist] (name removed) calling from Princess Margaret Hospital in Toronto. I'm just calling to see if you have arranged for any treatments locally. *We wouldn't want you to fall through the cracks now would we.* Please feel free to call me if you have any questions or if you would like to set up treatments up here. Ok Bye-bye now"

Fall through the cracks?! What the heck??!! I was not aware that I could potentially fall through the cracks - especially when I'm still looking for ANSWERS! Please, doc! You are the one who cast me aside ONE day like an old rotten tomato. You're the one who cancelled all the proposed upcoming tests that could have helped to properly diagnose my "stage" of cancer! This phone call just seems like a last-ditch effort - and a very lame one at that   -   to   relieve   your   conscience.

And THEN, if you can believe it, during my little afternoon nap the SAME day - I got another voicemail left for me....

"Hi Ken, this is Dr. [radiation oncologist] (name removed) I'm just following up with you because I see you have not really made any decisions regarding your treatments. I was just wondering if we could assist you in any way. Maybe through a PET scan or a biopsy of your lower lymph nodes? If you would like to talk about any of this further, I can be reached at...."

WHAT   THE   HECK??!!

The tests this doctor is talking about (the PET scan, etc...) are the SAME tests that were booked for me on May 14th (when the Toronto Docs thought I had stage 3 lung cancer). Those are also the SAME tests that were CANCELLED on me when the medical oncologist called me THE VERY NEXT DAY on May 15th to tell me that upon further review - they have changed their minds and do think I'm in stage 4.

I'm telling you - it's a REALLY good thing I have a sense of humour! I can't imagine how all this yo-yo-ing back and forth would mentally affect a 'terminal' cancer patient who was still depressed from hearing their diagnosis and prognosis. You would figure that these prestigious doctors at this world-renowned cancer hospital would have their 'poop'   together!   But   apparently   not.

My buddy Jim and I were joking on the phone yesterday afternoon comically imitating the doctors saying,

"Oh...So sorry Ken...you're gonna die now."
"Oh No... our mistake Ken! You're not dead yet - here's some hope."

"OOPS!! Did we give you hope yesterday? Sorry about that - we need that back"
"WAIT!! Here Ken! Here's some more hope we found on the floor in the corner"
"Our Bad! That wasn't hope - that was just a dust bunny...sorry. Just go home and die."

Like I said - at least I can laugh about it...

But yeah, I guess all this IS taking a toll on me but at least I can begin to see it from an outside perspective. I think part of the reason I'm able to 'step outside of myself' and laugh is because I don't believe one damn thing those big-shot doctors say anymore anyway. I believe in the healing power of God, and I believe in the power of Hope, Love, all of YOU and ME! I have decided to say; "To hell with the oncologists" - but there are others suffering out there that cannot or have not made that leap of faith. They don't know that there are other options. And I know...I KNOW that exactly what is happening to me, is happening to other people...and that's where my laughter changes to anger.

One of these days I'm gonna take my story public! To let other cancer sufferers out there know that they are being blindsided and 'herded" like cattle into a system whose only intent is to kill them slowly while making as MUCH money off them as they can in the process.

Sound a little callous?
Believe me - that IS what's going on! Big Pharmaceutical companies run the medical show folks. It's that simple.

Anyway, sorry to rant about this again - I just thought you all might like to know how the docs in Toronto are treating me. And PLEASE don't get me wrong...I'm NOT a doctor basher. There truly are wonderful physicians out there who actually care about their patients - and I'm lucky enough to know more than a few of them and am even honoured enough to call some of them 'friend'!

26
Voice for Choice
2007

In the meantime, Kenny googled other means of care, holistic, Reiki, supplements and natural. Radiation and chemotherapy have a 50/50 success rate if you call that successful.

Kenny's local oncologist wanted him to enter a trial experimental program she was conducting. He would die anyway because by now he was considered stage 4, but he would give her data for her research. Kenny said No and inclined toward alternative treatment. Through his father's advice, Kenny was driven twice a week across to Niagara Falls NY to Dr. Cutler for a treatment called "chelation" with a booster of vitamin C. Chelation was not recognized by the Canadian Medial Association, so the expense had to be paid for privately by Ken or Ken's family. Let's just say that this option drained the family's bank account.

29 May 2007 @ 7:44
Voice for Choice:
I'll tell you what I HAVE thought of doing though...and it involves the name I have mentioned in a few earlier posts: Voice for Choice™. Now I have already registered the domain name voiceforchoice.ca and in the near future when my cancer is further under control (or gone!) I would like to set up Voice for Choice™ as a charitable foundation

to help other people who are in the same boat that I am in right now. At this moment, as most of you know - I have been written off by the Canadian medical community and have been forced to research and find my own treatments elsewhere on the globe. Now, I have had TONS of help with that but just imagine if I was scared and all alone and didn't have all of you to draw on for support through my ordeal - where do you think would I be? Hey, I'm human! And being human, I'd probably be sitting on the nearest very tall bridge somewhere contemplating a jump, or at the very least have fallen into a DEEP depression! Well, Voice for Choice™ could change those feelings of emptiness and hopelessness.

I envision that this 'foundation' could offer (and I don't know how yet - I'm still working on it) counselling, support, financial aid, advice on 'alternative' treatment options and so much more to people and families that are fighting the same battle that we are.

*****

That blog written so many years ago reminds of Adam so much, with the human impulse to jump off a bridge if you are cornered with no option open to you for help. Adam, indeed, did just that a decade or so later. When Ford became Ontario Premier, things had not changed. Liberal, Conservative, whatever the stripe, things had not changed.

Kenny had to organize a fundraiser, held on Sunday June 24, at Beamsville Secondary School, so he could pay for his meds. The government was not forthcoming. Jim Gardner and his clothing company, Bruzer, out of Toronto, was the event's biggest sponsor, gathering prizes for a silent auction. The fundraiser was immensely successful raising thousands of dollars which, of course, disappeared within months gobbled up by the cost of Kenny's care. This event also saw Kenny launch his debut CD album of songs Kenny wrote himself and sang, called My Sentiments Exactly. Kenny expressed deep gratitude as I reread his Health Blog.

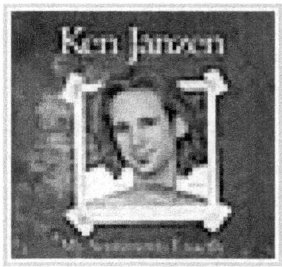

27
The Mulberry Bush

Round and Round he goes......
31. May 2007 @ 13:20

Sorry for the late posting today all! It was necessary as I had to go see my family doctor this morning. He had received...wait for it....
ANOTHER report from Princess Margaret Hospital (PMH) in Toronto and wanted me to see it and discuss it with me.

So, where we left off last time is that PMH had sent my family doctor a report the other week that turned out to be an old report with typos. (See the post from May 24th entitled "I'm What??!! AGAIN??!!" and the post from May 26th entitled "Is that a pogo stick? No, it's just Ken!" 😌

Well...here we go round the mulberry bush again! The radiation oncologist (the same one who left a voicemail last week) is the one responsible for this report. I will now quote some excerpts from the report - including the bad grammar and typos, followed by my own (quite cynical) responses.

"...on the basis that she [the medical oncologist] had at the time, it was not clear whether he [Ken] indeed has Stage 4 disease or not..."

Well duh! Why do you think I went to Toronto for a 2nd opinion??!!

"He [Ken] had multiple abnormalities within the left lung but some of them actually cleared on interval CT [catscan] and one of them on biopsy was not malignant."

Yeah - we knew about that. Conveniently forgot to mention my 2 shrinking lower lymph nodes though...

"...we had it [the CT scan of my abdomen] reviewed by a Radiologist *who very strongly felt* that this [my abdominal lymph nodes] is *likely* metastatic as there are no other obvious explanation for it."

Yeah...gee....no other reason...like...maybe...EPSTIEN BARR!!
How many 'drinks' did that Radiologist have at lunch before reviewing my scan anyway?

"Thus, we recommend that the patient commence radiotherapy and it seems *almost definitely* a Stage 4 disease and we feel that biopsy is warranted."

So, I'm "almost definitely" stage 4 (nice cover your butt wording there. doc) ...and yet NOW they feel a biopsy is 'warranted' - whereas 3 weeks ago they didn't??!

"If with time, the abdominal disease ends up being something else, then obviously the situation is different, and then aggressive treatment could be reconsidered."

Ya thinks??! Why do you think I wanted further tests done in the first place!

You have to know WHAT you are fighting in order to properly FIGHT it!

Sheesh!!! All I can say is that I'm getting pretty sick and tired of all this "up and down" crap.
Where did these guys get their medical degrees? Hollywood Upstairs Medical School?

OK...so to sum it all up, they have apparently changed their minds AGAIN - not about my staging (they are still assuming I am stage 4) - but NOW they have changed their willingness to offer different therapies - specifically radiation therapy and holy cow.... a biopsy! Wonders never cease!

Jeez...isn't THAT nice...NOW they feel that a biopsy is "warranted". Only after yanking my chain for what.... going on 3 weeks now??! And hmmmm.... lemme think a sec....isn't that what I've been asking for all along now...a biopsy of my lower lymph nodes to determine of the indeed are cancerous?

I will call the radiation oncologist back probably tomorrow and discuss the biopsy possibility with her. I also want to push for an MRI of the brain (to see if any cancer has spread there) and I'm REALLY gonna push for a PET scan (which will really help with my diagnosis). I may talk to the doctor about the radiation therapy as well - but seeing that the "mass" in my chest is right near my heart - undergoing radiation in that area can (and probably will) lead to some pretty serious damage to the heart muscle which can lead to a heart attack or something else down the road. Not sure if I like THAT idea...

But anyway, like I've said before - it's a good thing I have a healthy sense of humour and that I'm an emotionally strong person who has all of you to lean on - because if I was anything other than that right now - they'd probably have to lock me in a rubber room and just let me bounce around! (Some of you who know me well probably think I should be in a rubber room regardless - ha-ha)

BUT I know it is because of the sheer grace of God and your prayers and support - that we are getting through this. We are learning to handle the emotional ups and downs of all this much, much better than we had previously, partly because of my own sense of humour about all of this but mostly because of all of YOUR support! Again, we thank you and love you all!!! We can't say that enough!

I really don't know what's gonna happen next - all I can do is phone the doctor and push for the tests that I want done. And yes, don't fear, I'll keep you all in the loop - as always.

Felling a bit drained now - I should go and have some lunch...and then maybe my afternoon nap - or as my Opa used to call it (in German) ...my "Mittag Schlaf"!

Auf Wiedersehen for today all!

The Medical Mystery that is Me :) | Comments (11)

28
Channeled, Funneled
& Processed

Who knows if Kenny could have been saved if he had gone to the Saint Margaret Hospital in Toronto right away and if those faxes and reports between doctors would have been more quickly relayed and been followed up more quickly?

After a biopsy was finally done, the diagnosis was *"a poorly differentiated non-small cell adenocarcinoma"*. It's a form of lung cancer, they think. Kenny is very cynical about these non-committal answers.

"They are VERY clear in stating that it 'favours' or 'looks like' lung cancer…. which to me is well…. weird. The prudent thing to do is…if they truly don't know what it is or where it came from - then they should damn well find out!!!" [May 13, 2007]

Kenny thought the confusion could have come from the fact he also had *Epstein-Barr Syndrome*, a connection which the doctors never put together, nor pursued. Kenny felt cheated on the lack of further tests, and certainly all the delays in procedures. Valuable time passed by. May turned into June and June into July and July into August. Kenny was on heavy pain meds. By September, he was fed up. The title of one of his posts was: Answers? Who needs 'em! They finally got the answer they didn't want.

5 September 2007 @ 18:29
There's a "new" lymph node (new meaning that it was not affected before) just at the top of my stomach which is now approx. 8cm in diameter. THIS is the reason I have been in such severe pain and not able to sleep or eat. Honestly, it's just like Suzie said on our drive home from the doctors; between her sobs she said: "this is just like the first time we were told you had cancer. I thought that we would never have to go through that again".
"Me too hon!", I replied through my own sobs...."me too!"
And the sobs continue even now....

You know...I pray for help, and I get pain. I pray for food and sleep and that is kept from me. I pray for healing and of course, I am denied that as well - in fact a new tumour shows up. I don't know just how much more 'praying' I can take. What in the hell did I do to deserve this? So much for divine intervention.

Anyway, it looks like these past few months have NOT been stomach, digestive or ulcer problems, but the growth of that new tumour. And you know what? It's funny...you ask for tests, and they just give you medications.

In fact, I said this several times to the pain management nurse who was here last week. I DON'T want to take a new med "just because", I want to know WHY I need to take the med and what exactly the problem is that is causing me to take the med.

Medicine for the most part just masks the problem - it does not solve it!! If any of you out there ever have serious medical problems (and I hope NONE of you ever have to go through what I am) PUSH your doctor for tests, tests, and more tests to determine the actual problem, ask them to not just mask the solution with a quick flick of the pen on a prescription pad.

29
Time Drags On

Kenny was using pain patches and pills. By October, he was sent to Hamilton to add radiation to his therapy, which of course cured nothing. He had no more stamina. He could no longer blog. His sister, Marilyn, took over the job of "pinch-blogging".

OCTOBER 2007
Wanting but Can't :(
28. October 2007 @ 20:58
Well people, I am not Ken! I am his sister Marilyn. Kenny so desires to be back to blogging but does not have the energy or concentration to achieve it, yet! Kenny and Sue are so amazed at the number of people that have continued to comment even when he has not. Your comments, (and poems) warm his heart.

Checking the numbers and comments tonight, and the days when he can actually concentrate; brings such a warm smile to both Kenny and Sue.

So thank-you, from them and from the extended family for the out-pouring of your love through your writing.

Now an update on Kenny:

-Radiation has finished as of last Tuesday afternoon.
-He is HUNGRY! Praise God. He has gained over 10 pounds

since his radiation started. He was at 115 lbs.
but as of tonight, he is 125.5 lbs.

-The Dr's in Hamilton have started him on oral pills. They
will eventually ween him off the patch. He has no fat to
store the meds from the patches. (You would have
thought that the Dr's would have known that from day
one.)

-When he is up to it, he goes for a short walk outside with
Sue (around their circle). The fresh air does wonders for
him.

-Please continue to pray for healing, endurance, sleep, and
the feel of God's loving arms around him and his family.

Marilyn

*****

NOVEMBER 2007

The family was thinking of Christmas. What kind of
Christmas would it be? Kenny had a prayer list, not for
Santa but for his doctors:
Prayer list:
1) Sleep. He needs sleep so badly.
2) lower back pain is overpowering
3) Endurance to keep fighting this fight
4) the healing touch of God!
5) Please also pray for Sue.

Kenny was still hoping for a miracle but in November he
had lost a lot of weight. He looked like a pogo stick. He got
frustrated one evening while the family gathered around
the kitchen table. He yelled, "You don't understand!

You're not me!"   He shouted it out with a hoarse voice
that was constricted by cancer.

> Now listen to me, doctor, the business that you're in
> You must have seen a miracle time and time again
> If I can leave a number and the next one that you see
> If it ain't too much trouble, doctor, get in touch with
> me. *[Jesse Winchester song]*

DECEMBER 2007

Kenny was sleeping a lot. Whenever, the family would
visit during the autumn and winter months, little two-year-
old Braeden would always say, "Daddy sleeping." Marilyn
took over the chore of blogging. Kenny had no stamina.
Kenny's other sister, Marjorie [my wife] took over
comforting the kids or distracting them. Braeden was
often sent to Sue's mom.

Here is an excerpt from Bk. 1 of the trilogy, Time in a
Bottle, My brother-in-law got sick. Publ. on Amazon 2019.
* It should be noted that back in 2008, I asked Scott
Brettell for a copy of Kenny's Blog, since none of us were
handy with computers or thought to retain such a copy.
Scott thankfully obliged.

After Kenny's death, there was talk about writing a
book. Nothing was ever done. Traces of Kenny
disappeared off the internet, like little lights going out one
by one. After 11 years, I finally decided to write something
that could be published. Enough time had passed by. It
was difficult, despite the decade's passage of time, to
revisit the Blog. There was so much in the Blog, plus my
memories, that I came up with three books, not one. A

trilogy! Aptly entitled after Jim Croce's lovely song, "Time in a Bottle".

> If I could save time in a bottle
> The first thing that I'd like to do
> Is to save every day 'til eternity passes away
> Just to spend them with you

Kenny had a hankering for bacon and eggs. I said I'd make them for him, hoping that a bit of food would give him some strength. The smell of frying bacon filled the kitchen and that was soon filled with the smell of scrambled eggs. When was that? Back in November, December? Bk. 1, p. 297

I put some in a bowl for Kenny and took it downstairs. He only ate a bit and then poked around in the food. He still couldn't keep anything down. It was sad to see. "I'm sorry, Kenny." I wanted to see you eat.

Kenny got weaker and weaker. He was getting less steady on his feet. At one point, he tripped in the family room and crashed his head into the ornamental flashing around the fireplace putting a good dent into the copper framework.

30
Make it Stop!

We prayed that God would step in and do something to "Make it stop!" Make the pain stop, make the cancer go away. But it seemed like we were praying to empty space. Kenny was not rallying.

It was my chore to take Darriane out of the house, going for walks with her in the evening, the little 6-year-old, to get her out while the adults talked. I'd say, "Let's go visit your cousin, Cody." He lived a couple of blocks away and we'd have snowball fights on the way there. Darriane and I talked about the Christmas lights on the houses or how thick the snowflakes were.

I tried to write a poem, pleading with God: "If you will not take a prayer/ will you take a tear?" No other words came. No poem. My mind went numb. I felt God was too far away to listen, attending to distant galaxies, too busy planting the seeds of stars to pay attention to our family's needs...but I prayed anyway. Bk. 1, p.299

*****

Marilyn and Jerry stayed with Sue to talk around the kitchen table when Kenny slept downstairs in the hospital bed that had been brought in for him.

Kenny's father, Wally Janzen, wrote a few words close to Christmas on behalf of himself and the family.

A father's words!
20. December 2007 @ 18:47

Dear friends of Kenneth and Sue:

You may recall that several weeks ago Kenneth was scheduled to have a CT scan but didn't go because of feeling weak, etc. The scan was postponed until today but again they decided not to go which makes a great deal of sense to me. Kenneth is so drugged with morphine, hasn't slept for quite some time, hasn't really eaten much of anything, and is much too weak to make the long trek to Hamilton. Several months ago, the doctors told Kenneth and Sue that they would make that gradual change from morphine to methadone (it can't be done in one session) because morphine poses too many side-effects-it shuts down the bodily functions. Nothing was done for quite some time and now that his pain has surfaced again the only option is to give him more morphine. Kenneth rarely speaks and when he does it is in the form of a whisper. I believe he just doesn't have sufficient energy left to communicate.

Kenneth asked that we all meet at his house for our family Christmas dinner this coming Sunday. We are hoping and praying that he will be there with us to enjoy meeting some of the family who live at some distance and who haven't been able to see him and Sue as well as their little cousins   as   often   as   they   would   like. Over the years I have come to realize what a charismatic personality Kenneth has. His charm is so infectious and is evidenced by the many, many friends he has made. His blog and individual e-mails directed to me have told me time and again how much he is loved by so many. Sue read Ed Warneck's blog comments to him. When I asked him whether he knew that Ed had commented, a great big smile crossed his face. This was sufficient proof how much he had appreciated your words, Ed. I find it extremely difficult to think that God knows best in all instances and especially for my son. He is loved so dearly by the family, and his immediate family needs him so very much. I have read all the prayers that you have posted on his blog, and it appears that God chooses to answer as He chooses. (The pot does NOT dictate to the Potter how it is to be made and what its function is and how long it is to be used. I realize that I am selfish and only want what I think is best for my son whom I love so dearly.)

In the months that Kenneth has had to endure his illness, he has never really complained. Had he had the stamina he would have told all of you repeatedly how much you have meant to him, how much your comments on this blog have provided emotional support for him and Sue. He appreciated you being there for him and his extended family.

Sue has had a heavy load to bear over these months as you can well imagine.
Please continue to pray for Kenneth, Sue, Darriane, and Braeden.

Thank you to all who have been so supportive, empathetic, and compassionate.

Sincerely,
Wally (dad)

The Medical Mystery that is Me :) | Comments (41)

Re: A father's words!
By Marjorie
22. December 2007 @ 18:13

It's been quite a while since I last posted. John keeps up with the Blog, but I find it too hard to read and I end up sobbing. John showed me Dad's letter tonight as I was wrapping Christmas presents for Darriane and Braeden and after the tears dried, I reached for my Bible and opened it to a passage that I have underlined and have read many, many times this year. It's Psalm 42, specifically verse 11.

Why am I discouraged? Why so sad? I will put my hope in God! I will praise him again - my Savior and my God! Medicine cannot cure Kenny, doctors seem unable to help much, there's nothing we can do but pray and be there for Kenny and our family.

Only God can change the situation. It's in His Hands. Kenny, Sue, Darriane, and Braeden, you are all so special to us. We love you so! We continue to pray!

Marjorie.

31
Christmas

Kenny rallied enough on Christmas Day to post. I decided to keep all the typos as a picture of the disoriented state he was in because of his meds. Yet, the fire of his intelligence comes through.

The Prodical Son returns this Christmas day!
25. December 2007 @ 08:10
HEY ALL!!! MERRY CHRISTMAS TO ALL OF YOU!!!!

I have missed chatting at you all so, so, much, And it has been a heavy burden wearing on my soul that I find it hard to blog every day like I used to. The medication I'm onm still makes it VERY hard for me to focus and type - it even makes it difficult to dictate to someone else, becase you tend to forget where your pointt was going.

Anyway what better day that the birthday of our Lord Jesus Christ could I pick to try my weary hand at blogging once again?

And know this...even thouhg I have not been posting for the last few months, i HAVE been reading and your comments are simply....glorious, uplifting and so much more that mere words can describe. THey have definately been a source of fuel and lova for me cna ny family and a lot of other folks out there and for that again I can only say thank-you.

Come to think of it, I find it amazing what my little blog has turned into this past year and I'm sure it will metaphorphasize again into other even more positive things

Well, the kids will be getting up soon and thianks to tje generousity of SO many people -, there are so may gifts undeer the tree for my two womderful kids, that it has just simply made me sit here and weep - because months earlier I didn't know how we would even be able to "Do" Christmas this year. And once again, just when you think all is lost, manna appears from heaven in the form of presents for my two amazing little kids. Thanks you Lord!!!!!!! And thank you to all of you who have given so generouersouly and selflessly of yourselves to us this season - we could NOT have done it wothout you this year.

OOPS. I think I hear little feet starting to stir - I better run. We love you all!
So Merryy Christmas to all of you, spelling mistakes and all

Till the next time (which will be soon...I promise)
I lova each and every one of you,
Ken

The Medical Mystery that is Me :) | Comments (56)

32
New Year's 2008

There was nothing to celebrate on New Year's 2008. We knew we would lose Kenny. I do not know if MAiD, which was legalized in Canada, only 8 years later, in 2016, would have made a difference to Kenny. He kept on fighting to the very end, even when he slipped into a coma during the last three days of his live. He had so much to live for. He was only 37 years old! Marilyn kept "pitch-blogging" for her brother, Kenny.

*****

New Day!
7. January 2008 @ 18:07

-Kenny is on oxygen now most of the time. That started Sat. Jan. 5 around 4 am. He felt he could not breathe well enough on his own. There have been times when he takes it off, but only for a short spell.

-He has been trying to eat. Sunday morning, he was asking for bacon and eggs. Now he has not really eaten anything in the last few weeks. Sue felt that maybe cream of wheat might be easier on his stomach. He ate half. (The bowl was not that full)

-He is having difficulty getting his pills down. He feels that they are getting stuck.

-He is also unstable on his feet.

-He fell Sunday afternoon, & he hit his head on the side of the fireplace. That was a major scare for Sue and me. No bleeding, and nothing was broken. He does have a hard head.   🙂

The family has been HANGING out at Kenny and Sue's. Kenny has been wondering why we are always there. Each time he opens his eyes we still seem to be there. "We just like spending time with you and your family" is what we tell him! The family has gone back to work today so his house should have been quieter.

Marilyn.

The hardest Journey
13. January 2008 @ 09:12

Thank you to all of our blogger family for being with us through this journey. This journey we are taking is a hard one. We have never walked this walk before and wish to never walk it again. This past week has been a very hard one. Unless you have had a loved one struggle with cancer you really do not know what we are experiencing. This past week Marjorie and I took days off of work to spend with Kenny and Sue. Even Andrew (my youngest) stayed one night and all of the next day to help. Kenny and Andrew have this special bond that is beyond just Uncle and Nephew. When you see them together, you almost feel like crying. Andrew holds Kenny in his arms and talks. Just talks about anything & everything. And Kenny is listening and trying to hold Andrew back. We are making sure that Sue is never alone. Our family is there to support and comfort Sue, play, and occupy Darriane and take care of Kenny. This past week has been called "Family Week". Sue understands that friends are wishing to drop by for a visit. We are at the stage of Kenny's life where Kenny does not visit anymore. Kenny's day consists of sleeping, we wake him up for his meds (which might take up to 2 hours for us to get into him), hopefully a bathroom break and then back to sleep. He seems to be pain free. Sue has picked up liquid Methadone just in case the swallowing becomes too hard.

The other morning, Sue and I checked the blog map to see where all of the bloggers are coming from. WOW, you are around the world. That is so amazing. We also noticed that Kenny had over 7200 blogger hits for the month of Dec/07. 2900 of those bloggers are from St. Catharine's alone. You are our neighours and are showing us, you care and are praying. Thank you so very much. The family does feel your prayers. Right now, that is almost all that you can do. Friends and extended family are asking "what can I do for you? Just give me a call!". Praying right now for peace and strength is everything.

To Kenny's and Sue's friends: please keep calling them. Sue needs to know that you are still with her and caring. Every time a friend calls, she tells Kenny you called, and he tries to smile. They need your calls, please don't stop. One day Kenny might be up for a visit with you, but most times he is sleeping.

To our blogger family: please keep posting. Sue has been checking a few times each day, to read any new comments. They are helping her to get through each day. Again, thank you for your prayers. They have been felt like a comforting fuzzy blanket around us. If you have not read John's comment from yesterday, please go back and read it. This is our family. We are a very close & loving family.

Lovingly
Marilyn.

33
Night and Day

Re: The hardest Journey by John and Marjorie
14. January 2008 @ 22:32

Timelessness
In the beginning God created
the heavens and the earth.
the earth was without form,
and void; and darkness was on
the face of the deep. And the
Spirit of God was hovering over
the face of the waters. *Gen. 1:1*

Ken's days are the same as his nights. Everything blends together in drugged timelessness. Ken is afraid of the dark, so the TV above the fireplace is on all the time, tuned either to cartoons or to decorating shows. The lights in the room are also on, set with the dimmer switch. We are lucky that the washroom is just a short shuffle down the hallway. Ken's nights and days are reduced to simple functions. Sleep, meds, washroom, sleep.

It's not a healing sleep. We all know this is different. Ken's computer downstairs in his office sits unused, the monitor lit on screensaver. How we all wish that Ken would wake tomorrow, healed, and new, and ready to fire up his programs for another website design.

But it's not so, and the only comfort we can extend now is to just be there. It's not good to ask too many questions. That irritates him. Ken takes minutes to respond to even one question. And our time is not his time, whether he has to sit up finally for his meds or to lie back down so his feet can be lifted up on the couch by somebody.

He needs a helping hand with everything. Even a Kleenex is hard to control, an end held with one hand and fingers fumbling gingerly and missing the edge of the other end so he can't stretch it to blow his nose. Family is there to help, even to readjust the Kleenex in his hands.

The Medical Mystery that is Me :) | Comments (17)

A spoonful of pudding....
15. January 2008 @ 08:25

BEFORE I REPORT IN....PLEASE GO BACK TO YESTERDAYS COMMENTS. EACH ONE WILL MELT YOUR HEART AND I KNOW WILL BRING TEARS TO YOUR EYES.

Part of me finds it difficult to write about Kenny's last few days. Our family is allowing you to share in our struggles, our tears, our smiles, our prayers, and our love for Kenny. You are able to walk beside us,
and hold us up in prayer as only close friends can. With each few words that I type, I must stop and wipe away the tears for I cannot see the keyboard anymore. This is so hard for us.

I must tell you that Kenny is still fighting. He has not given up completely. His body is saying goodbye, but his mind still tries to focus. I stayed with Sue Sunday night and around 2 am, we woke Kenny up for his meds. I had the TANG (which was/is favourite orange drink) with a straw and Sue had the chocolate pudding and meds. (This is all the nourishment we get into him.) Sue was giving him his spoonful of pudding with 1 pill, then a spoonful of pudding without. We are using baby spoons. Kenny tried to tell us something which we could not understand. We asked 3-4 times "pardon me, can you repeat it Kenny?" Finally, he was so annoyed with us that he very slowly but with much umph... said," alternate, juice, pudding, juice, pudding, juice, pudding, GOT IT?" Sue and I laughed. We got it. We told him that we will never forget it now. We were told.
☺

After that the meds went down smoothly, now we knew how he wanted it. We asked him if he wanted to lay back down to rest. He shook his head. What do you do at 2:30 in the morning? So, I talked. I told him stories about each one of my children, their spouses, my grandchild, about Jerry, and just rambled on and on until 4-ish. Then he said he was ready to sleep. Every so often during my talking, he would nod or mouth WOW, so we knew he needed that time with us. That will stay with me for the rest of my life. Monday afternoon, Kenny became despondent. He would not acknowledge anything. We tried for over 2 hours.... nothing. From our special time to this.... The family MD stopped in for a house visit last night, at Sue's request. Kenny's eyes are glazed over, and Kenny complains he cannot see anymore. His lungs according to the MD are fine. ??????

Marjorie stayed Monday night and Jerry & I went home around 10pm. Andrew came for a visit last night. Kenny needed to be woken up around 9:30 so Andrew was allowed to wake him. Andrew held the juice while Sue did the meds. Andrew started singing...."A spoonful of pudding helps the Methadone go down, the Methadone go down, the Methadone go down, just a spoonful of pudding helps the Methadone go down, In the most delightful way!" Kenny started to smile and actually swayed to Andrews singing. Now for us watching.... We wanted to shout Thank You Andrew, and cry at the same time. Andrew had Kenny smiling and responding. Andrew stayed till 12, until Kenny was ready to sleep. Marjorie called me this morning to let me know that the night was peaceful. His feet/legs are still very swollen and cold, his hands are cold now also. Most times he does not open his eyes. We cherish each smile,
and each "I love you" that comes from our brother.

For the people that have not experienced this walk with a family member, you are living it now through us.

Marilyn

ADDITION   :
I have been constantly talking to you about our family and our journey that we are on. But I feel like I must ask for forgiveness from Sue's family. They have been walking this journey right along with Sue. They see Sue struggling to be strong each day and people feel for her. They feel helpless without knowing what to do. The family is in close contact with Shirley daily for her to pass on loving remarks to Sue

and Kenny. To our blogger family: please continue to pray for Sue's side also. For there are 2 sides to every family.

*****

The Medical Mystery that is Me :)|Comments (71)

Re: A spoonful of pudding....by Wally Janzen
15. January 2008 @ 09:37

William H. Davies, America's educated hobo poet wrote these lines: "And no man dies, but must look back, with sorrow on his own past track." A week or so ago, Kenneth told Sue that his concern was that God would say, when he arrives at heaven's door, "And why should I let you in. It was only when you became ill that you returned to me. And now you want in?" Sue relayed this apprehension to us, and I spent some time assuring Kenneth that God does not keep score. Jesus has done EVERYTHING for us; there is nothing we can do to deserve or earn our heavenly home. I tried to reassure him that the Bible is so very consistent regarding this message to us. It talks about the thief on the cross, who just hours before his death, and so undeserving of any mercy was told that he and Jesus would be together in paradise. And then I told Kenneth about the parable in Matthew 20 where the employer hires workers at various times throughout the day but remunerates them the same. (I love this story.) But the parable that has had the greatest impact on me is that of the Prodigal Son. Regardless of his past misdeeds, his father loved him enough to wait for his return EVERY DAY without fail. And who can forget the Good Shepherd who leaves his ninety-nine sheep in order to search for the one that was/is lost.

God has provided these stories for our assurance of salvation if we believe that Jesus truly is God's Son. I am so appreciative of my family that we are able to band together to support not only Kenneth and Sue but that we are there for one another in good times as well as those times that are most difficult. You are loved so much! And, thank you to all (readers of the blog and friends) who have been and are so very supportive. Please continue in prayer for Kenneth and his family. Wally (dad)

34
Letting Go

Going over the Blog this evening so many years later, in 2023, was too much for me. I took my e-bike out at 8:30 pm, to bounce the basketball off the church wall. It was cool after the evening rain. I enjoyed it. I noticed a little, white moth on the brick wall, so I kept to the left of it to bounce the ball. "Leave it alone," I thought, "it's not in my clothes closet." The little beastie must have clung on for the last radiating heat from the afternoon sun. If it shoved off the wall, who knows what cruel elements it would have flown into in the cooling evening air.

I came home to make peppermint tea for my wife and then made a beehive for my office and my computer. "Buffy, the Vampire Slayer," was doing an artsy musical singsong with Spike and the rest of the vampire gang. I'm not into vampire musicals. Besides, Buffy was not a good enough singer to catch my attention.

I remember January 2008, the last 18 days of Kenny's life. MAiD was not available then. Would he have chosen it? Would he have said, I can't make my family go through this; I can't make myself go through this? He was still fighting for his connection to the world. He was still in his 30s, for Pete's sake!

I still think of what could have been, should have been, might have been but wasn't. Kenny had been in a coma for 3 days. Who knows what he dreamed of, in what realm his mind moved. I wrote something in the Blog about

Comas and Choices. I imagined Kenny living out his life in his coma to a ripe old age.

To see a world in a grain of sand
And heaven in a wildflower
Hold infinity in the palm of your hand
And eternity in an hour.
   -- from 'Auguries of Innocence'
     William Blake (1757 - 1827)

I thought I was being profound. It didn't matter.

*****

Kenny took his last breath on January 18, 2008, at 3:39 p.m. The oxygen reader read 0. Dad was heard to utter, "My boy. My boy."

When Kenny breathed his last, the family physician was called. He made a house call.

Tallman Funeral Home showed up with a van and a gurney. The burden was light. We stood by crying. Winter, cold, snow outside. We silently turned our minds to God and asked: Why?

Some will win, some will lose
Some were born to sing the blues
Oh, the movie never ends
It goes on and on and on and on
  (*Journey*, Don't Stop Believing, 1981)

Time for
a cool change...
I know that it's time
for a cool change
  (Little River Band 1979)

35
One Day at a Time

One Day at a Time
February 2008 @ 13:08

I'm not sure where to begin, but I thought it was about time that I blogged and express my sincere thanks to everyone who has commented, sent a card, flowers etc. Every written letter and hug were always appreciated, along with people providing meals for our family. Probably everyone is wondering how I am doing. Before Ken passed away, I would always tell people that I take it a day at a time. That is still my answer when people ask me. When Ken passed away, there were funeral arrangements and decisions that had to be made, (thank you to my family for making that job easier), then the viewings along with the funeral. I have still been pretty busy after the funeral with paperwork and more paperwork and trying to get my life organized and take care of the children. Braeden doesn't understand too much and asks where daddy is once in a while. We always say daddy is in heaven now. Darriane is dealing with it pretty well with some emotional outbursts once in a while. We are looking into grieving counseling for myself and as well as for Darriane. There are times when I'm alone that I will let go of my feelings, but I still have a pretty tough wall up. I'm having a hard time breaking it down. I go through a roller coaster of feelings ranging from being scared to feeling numb. I have been looking at pictures and remembering the fun times we had and all the dreams we were some days hoping to fulfill. Even the little things that Ken held dear to his heart mean the world to me.

There have been many people sharing their feelings with me, letting me know that Ken is very much here in spirit. It's nice to know that others feel him around them as well and I'm not the only one talking out loud to him as if he was standing in front of me. I really do feel him around me and there has been strange things happening - like hearing our songs together, a t-shirt that was the only one there staring at me that read "Snowflakes and kisses sent from heaven", our wedding song on the radio and his little voice inside my head joking with me. People probably will think that I'm looking for things to remind me of him – which may be true, but I prefer to think that he is sending me little messages and I don't want to miss one message from him.
P.S. I will try to keep the blog going for everyone. Sue.

| Comments (82)

*****

P.P.S. by John: Even the blog fizzled out. There were no more postings or comments. There was no more Ken. There was nothing really to keep the Blog going.

36
It's Been 15 Years!

Kenny was pretty well grounded in reality, loving what was honest and good and hating what was empty and full of lies. In his office/man-cave, Kenny imbibed the music of groups like *Journey, Sting, Toto,* and *Econoline Crush*, who sang about hope, dreams, love, loneliness, and the search for lasting values:

> *Momentary fashion, the passing of a phase*
> *Calculated drivel from empty soul parade*
> *Pabulum for the masses, you can't dig the grave*
> *All you ever wanted was a little piece of fame*
> *Oh your lies.*
> *Lies (*Econoline Crush "Sycophant" 1995)

It's 2023 now. Full-fledged summer. There are 482 wildfires in Canada. My wife and I drove into St. Catharine's for grocery shopping on Wednesday and everything was hazy. Smog from the fires. The smoke has even reached Europe and the U.S. newspaper headline reads, Blame Canada!

It's been 15 years since Kenny's death. Sue has remarried and Braeden and Darriane are almost young adults. Nobody wants to revisit those painful months, weeks, and days in 2008 when Kenny lay dying. Life goes on. Yet, for my part, since I'm a writer, I'd like to leave evidence of him in my books. He was an amazing person.

I copied Kenny's websites onto DVDs, also adding a copy of his Blog. I intended to give these copies to Braeden and Darriane when they got older. But they wouldn't be interested in these things now. Life demands concentration on the present, not a visit to a melancholy past. Forget, forget, forget, whatever is painful and sad!

When we sell the house and move to a condo, I will probably throw these DVDs away. That would be Kenny's wish as well, to let his kids go do their own thing in life, to set them free of the past, like butterflies.

*****

Kenneth Wayne Janzen was buried in the Vineland Old Mennonite cemetery. During that January and February of 2008, I felt I needed to resolve something. I did not know what. The answer to life? To death?

I visited Kenny's Grave several times those slushy winter days, galoshes on, a winter coat and gloves. It was cold and damp. I stared at the marker, no gravestone yet. I trudged home and wrote a poem.

My wife says that Kenny would not have used MAiD. He would have fought, like the eye of the tiger [*Survivor*], to the very end, hoping either for a cure through a persistent battle with natural meds or for a miracle.

If he would have used MAiD, it would have been just after Christmas when his body was failing. After Christmas, he had just over 3 weeks to live, the way he was going. MAiD could have saved him much pain and a final coma. At least, he would have had Christmas with the family.

37
Renate Hartig

My sister, Renate, affectionately called Reni, died on July 3, 2016, at the age of 67 after a long battle with Multiple Sclerosis.

She had suffered from the disease for 20 years, slowly enduring its onslaught against her fine motor functions, her balance, mobility, vision, and memory.

Ironically, she died the same month and year that MAiD was legalized. Since she died in early June, however, she could not have taken advantage of MAiD with the process of application and then the waiting period which took time. She had no choice but to let nature take its course.

Even if she had a choice, I don't think she would have taken it. The red tape would have been too involved, since a patient had to be approved by two independent physicians or nurse practitioners, and then there was, of course, that waiting period. Besides, she was brought up Catholic and thought suicide, in any form, was wrong.

Since 2016, euthanasia has become Canada's sixth leading cause of death. Currently, there are many critics about the use of MAiD, saying that its parameters have extended too far to also include the irremediably mentally ill, not just the terminally ill!

Multiple Sclerosis attacks myelin, the covering of the nerves, causing inflammation and obviously destroying the functioning of the nerve. Often there is recovery and then regression, toying with a person's hope, like one step forward and two steps back. A person has tingling, bladder problems, cognitive impairment, and mood changes. It's a sad disease, indeed with no cure. If there is a God, it's one of his cruel punishments upon mankind.

Canada has one of the highest rates of MS in the world. An estimated 90,000 Canadians live with the disease. Most people are between the ages of 20 and 49. My sister first had symptoms when she was 46 years old where she fumbled with the dishes in the kitchen, dropped things, tripped over things, and kept falling down the stairs.

We assume that other people are healthy like we are, when we ask them how they are. We expect an automatic response of "Fine", and then we go our way. We don't see hidden problems in their lives, nor care to hear them.

The family thought my sister was just clumsy. Her family went through a traumatic time once the real cause for her clumsiness was discovered.

When her disability got bad enough, my sister went into the Trinity Seniors' Home in Kitchener. This was ironic in that my mother, Rosa, was there too in her old age. Mom was 93 when she died in the home. She stopped eating; her body atrophied. I wonder if someday MAiD might intervene in these homes to give clients in a coma the needle to hurry death along, thinking that this act would be a mercy, to put the patient to sleep, instead of letting nature take its course.

Anyway, my sister, Reni, was still quite young, in her late 50s, when she went into the home. At least, she and mom could visit each other. They also had Nick, who visited regularly. Reni had met him in the hospital when she broke a bone.

We value people depending upon their individual gifts, their education, and their personality, also their experiences and history. Reni had a good job after graduating from St. Mary's High School, becoming secretary to Kitchener's mayor at the old City Hall.

This was a respectable accomplishment for the daughter in a refugee family who had immigrated to Canada from Austria in 1954, shortly after WW II with two suitcases to their name.

Reni was 5 at the time; I was 8. I still remember living in the army barracks in Austria, barracks that had been abandoned by the Nazis after the Allies won the war. Living conditions were poor. Dad applied to come either to Canada or Australia to create a new life with the help of the Lutheran church. The application for Canada came through.

Kitchener at the time was going gangbusters with construction. I remember how rich these Canadians seemed, with their black and white TVs and their Christmas trees. I wore my lederhosen to school in grade 1 and was called a Nazi, a DP, and beaten up by 5 Polish kids. Breaking into the new culture was tough until we learned the language. I don't recall that my sister was harassed, maybe because she started out younger, at age 5. I remember absorbing the culture with heroes on TV like the Lone Ranger and Robin Hood.

My sister, I know, absorbed the music of teenage idols like Frankie Avalon and Ricky Nelson. I remember dad watching Hockey Night in Canada in the basement when Foster Hewitt would yell, He Shoots. He scores!

Citizenship is such an ephemeral thing, sometimes the accidental byproduct of a war.

38
Our Background

My father Michael was born in Romania in a German speaking village named Teckendorf. This was in the province of Transylvania. Queen Maria Teresa had invited these Saxons, in the 18th century, known for their farming, forestry and mining skills, into that region of the Austro-Hungarian Empire to make it prosper, and they did! Dad's father, Johann, was a miller who had a business grinding grain for the farmers around the Teckendorf area.

Mom, Rosa, came from a region along the Danube River which is now Serbia. She could speak 5 languages, like my dad. Her original home was Alsace Lorraine which always bounced back and forth between Prussia and France. She was part of a Germanic group known as Donau-Schwabians, Donau meaning the Danube River.

When WW II broke out, the Russians did not make the fine distinction between Germans, Saxons and Donau-Schwabians. Anybody caught behind the Russian lines was either murdered or sent to Siberia. Mom and Dad's families fled to Austria, specifically settling in abandoned German army barracks near Linz. These barrack communities originally housed German soldiers. When the Allies won, they housed DPs, displaced persons and families who left their lands and farms behind in the hands of Communist Russia.

A community of barracks was called a "Lager", meaning camp. The Americans numbered these camps. Our camp, outside of Linz, was number 67. Every nationality of

Europeans could be found in a camp, all displaced people with nothing to their names. I remember our family getting CARE packages from the U.S. army. An American army chaplain, Mr. Ackerman, would drive into Lager Wegscheid with his jeep and give my parents a CARE package and something extra at Christmas time, because my name was on their list as a baby with rheumatic fever and tuberculosis. I remember that these Yanks were known for two things, chocolates and chewing gum.

Thanks to the Marshall Plan, Europe was being rebuilt after the war. But in the late 40s and early 50s, we had not benefited from a rebuilt Europe yet. Some of the Hartigs emigrated to Australia. We came to Canada. Dad became enamored with hockey. We became Canadians. Mom and Dad loved old John Diefenbaker, Canada's Prime Minister from 1957 to 1963.

*****

My wife's history too, as Mennonites, traced its ancestry back to Ukraine where they built productive farms and where they lost everything in the Russian Revolution of 1917. Mennonites were accepted as refugees throughout the 1920s in Canada, to farm the poor soils of Saskatchewan's prairies to start all over. They left the prairies, uprooted themselves once more in the 1940s and moved to Ontario's Niagara Peninsula and the fecund farmlands of orchards and flowers. Mennonites became successful again, strengthened by their religion and a firm work ethic. They built houses and churches and were prosperous citizens in Canada because they had a cooperative community, and they knew how to work.

Somehow, I think that modern immigrants to Canada have it easier. Mostly coming from the Middle East and mostly flying over on jet planes.

We came by boat in 1954 crossing the Atlantic Ocean on the S.S. Neptunia in the tumultuous November storms. We were seasick. The train ride by steam locomotive was arduous chugging across Quebec Province until we stepped off at the Kitchener train station with our two suitcases.

Dad got work on construction as a laborer and then learned how to drive the forklift which brought buckets of mortar to bricklayers.

*****

We were grateful when Canada brought in its Universal Healthcare system in the 1960s to take care of its own citizens when they needed surgery and expensive medical care.

Canada has come a long way in adopting social programs even for new immigrants to provide housing, education, and healthcare, when in the 1950s much of that was not there for new people.

It's been a wonderful country for my family. I went to university and have become a writer. But as we grew to love Canada in the old days, we did not know what lay ahead. We did not know there could be a recession even here in Canada. Nor a housing shortage, nor homelessness, nor the fact that 1 out of 9 students go to school hungry, nor a failing healthcare system.

Nor the side effects of a Pandemic from 2019 to 2022 where seniors died in their own feces in old folks' homes in Ontario, where the army had to be called in to help out, and where our Premier Doug Ford refused to hire more healthcare workers.

We also did not know about MAiD, nor whether this kind of mercy killing was good or bad for society. One thing for sure, it is cost effective!

Instead of spending the money to keep people alive, with programs, counseling, surgeries and meds; it's quicker to give them a needle to kill them.

*****

I had a recent heart incident in September 2023, at the age of 77. Arrythmia which nearly killed me. I've got an ICD implanted in my chest now, a combination defibrillator and pacemaker. Mind you, tax money paid for it, but in the follow-up, when I asked about counseling and psychiatric help, because I've been feeling down lately since my dangerous heart incident, administration wanted to know if I had, insurance, or the money to cover the cost for such extended psychological care.

The whole system is geared to shaking more money out of you at the end of your life. Capitalistic forces know where the cracks are to destroy the socialistic, universal healthcare which we so cherished, so that private for-profit interests, fueled by greed, can destroy the socialistic system that Tommy Douglas and Lester Pearson originally championed for all Canadian citizens regardless of income. A respectable system was, indeed, achieved and enjoyed for many years...and over the past few decades, because of greedy companies from within Canada and powerful capitalists from the United States, right next to us, our universal system has been dealt death blows and transformed into "for-profit" private health companies they have in the United States!

This is most evident in Ontario, where our Premier, Doug Ford, has been subleasing minor surgeries like cataracts and even knee surgeries to the private sector to ease wait times.

Doug Ford's motives are questionable. Let's ignore the Greenbelt scandal for a moment. Let's look at his healthcare track record since the Pandemic.

The Liberal government subcontracted not only cataract and knee surgeries to private companies but also hip and even heart surgeries. This is all in the name of creating a hybrid system to make wait times better for everybody. But in reality what has it done? It's opened the floodgates to private healthcare in Canada for those who have money!

*****

Two-tier, three-tier care is implanted into our current system and people are being billed extra for it! Tommy Douglas and Universal Healthcare ideals are history! I will never forget the many seniors who died in for-profit homes during the Pandemic because Doug Ford refused to hire more staff. The army had to be called in to clean up the mess and care for the seniors who were dying in their own feces.. How shameful!

That is why MAiD is going to expand its parameters by March 2024 to include the mentally ill, as another cost cutting tactic for the government. It's cheaper to kill the problem, than to keep suffering people alive! Euthanasia does not save lives; it saves money! Money, not mercy, is the driving force behind MAiD?

I admit that the problem is not clearcut, that there are difficult moral boundaries. Certainly, in some cases, there could be no relief where there is no cure, other than to put someone out of their misery. But what if the government did have the money to provide programs, more medical staff and meds for suffering people whose lives might still be productive if, and only if, there was that money and staff available to make their lives easier?

We are faced with two questions. First, how do we take care of our citizens in a universal healthcare system that does not fail? And secondly, how do we administer MAiD in a truly humane and merciful way to only those who suffer where it's necessary?

39
MAiD's Future

As the mandate in MAiD redefines its parameters, the question about its morality is still up in the air. I suppose it makes sense when there is no escape from terminal sickness if you are in inescapable pain. You have to go sometime, so make the process of death when it is a professional and painless process, like going to sleep. Although nobody may admit it, the process is also a cost-effective choice for the government. Critics say that life could be prolonged in comfort if the government spent money for it.

I can see MAiD popping up like service stations within our cities, usually next to hospitals and "health centers". That certainly would relieve pressures off hospitals and seniors' homes. There will be a proliferation of funeral homes too, more services offered, and more cemeteries and crematoriums built. It will become a burgeoning business.

I don't like the idea. However, after Matt's experience and also Adam's, I said to my wife, if I ever get to the point of drooling in my wheelchair in a seniors' home, suffering from dementia, put me out of my misery with MAiD. That is no quality of life. Cremate me and be done with it.

We have had a happy life together and good memories to share, but if I get a terminal disease and a mind that is gone, I do not want the family to endure long months of suffering. It's not healthy to pass such pain along to my loved ones, and it's not fair.

Canada reached a milestone in 2023 in its population, exceeding 40 million people spread over this large land, mostly clustered in the big cities of Montreal, Toronto, and Vancouver. New immigrants proliferate in those centers. It's okay for Prime Minister Trudeau to say he wants to bring in another 24,000 immigrants from the Middle East, but the government needs to be sensible, that it is able to provide the programs to take care of and assimilate these people. The system is going to break, not able to take care of the citizens that already live here. Seniors' homes are short staffed. Nurses are overworked. Doctors too don't like the changes in the failing system.

In the meantime, our Mosaic of Canada is fracturing, with indigenous demands for reconciliation, and probably more money from Ottawa, LGBTQ demonstrations, protests against the police, and on the macrocosmic level, Quebec wanting its independence, the Prairies also not happy with Ottawa, and British Columbia seeing itself separate because of the Rockies.

We are indeed a shaky Confederation! 157 years old this July 1, 2023. Meanwhile, Ottawa is renovating its Parliament buildings to the tune of 5 billion dollars, while healthcare goes private, and the country has rumors of its healthcare system falling apart.

Maybe the country needs its own kind of MAiD to put all its economic ailments out of its misery? How will we be reborn to overhaul ourselves into a decent standard of living? We don't even have a clear identity as a country!

Unfortunately, politicians align with party lines and do not fight for what is sensible and good for the whole. There is a self-destruct mechanism in the human psyche which is dark.

*****

Mark Twain once joked about the human psyche, saying that he was not a pessimist, he was merely an optimist who had not arrived. Somehow, he saw countries and politicians muddling along from one generation to the next, forever conspiring to hold onto power. Somehow, they always survive, don't they! Despite all that mess, we need men and women of good conscience, who will bring us to a better place, who will fight for the best for all. There are such people! Thomas Jefferson, Abraham Lincoln, John Diefenbaker, Lester Pearson. There is also the dark side, Adolph Hitler, Idi Amin, and Vladimir Putin. We must be a light in the darkness. Democracies have some good ideas. Despots are greedy. Machiavelli wrote The Prince, a great handbook for a despot who puts the population down and uses people for the self-aggrandizement of the ruling class. Some countries still are not beyond that kind of thinking, oppressed by their leaders.

Hitler had "social programs" for eliminating people who were not productive in society. Gypsies, Jews, the mentally deficient, the lame and the unemployed. We must make sure that our enlightened democratic society does not have MAiD expand its parameters to embrace programs which align with the dark side of getting rid of people. Let's hope our Supreme Court Justices are equal to the task.

For what is one life worth? Economists say a human life is worth about $10 million. Or is it invaluable as religious people say? I am touched by the lyrics in the musical, "Rent". "The Seasons of Love" enumerates the days and minutes in a life.

Five hundred twenty-five thousand, six hundred minutes
Five hundred twenty-five thousand moments so dear
Five hundred twenty-five thousand, six hundred minutes
How do you measure, measure a year?

In daylights, in sunsets
In midnights, in cups of coffee
In inches, in miles
In laughter, in strife
In five hundred twenty-five thousand, six hundred minutes
How do you measure a year in the life?

How about love?
How about love?
How about love?
Measure in love
Seasons of love...
Remember the love.

40
W5, Canada's News Watchdog

Canada has some great news documentaries which keep its citizens informed about controversial topics, about things wrong with our society and about how things need to change. W5 and Marketplace have spread awareness to the Canadian public for decades about hot topics. The problem is, once said or pointed out, does the system actually act upon it. Where are the politicians and the people in a position to change what's wrong? And if there is change, who is to make sure that the change is done correctly...and morally!

W5 aired an episode in July 2023 on MAiD's intention to expand its mandate to people who are mentally ill. That episode was aired just over half a year before the new law to include the mentally ill was to go into effect in March of 2023.

John Scully, 81: "I've had enough of this. It was just a cold, simple decision. I've got to stop this and the only way to stop this was to kill myself." He tried to overdose in 2006 but the wife called 911 and rescued him. He had his stomach pumped. He's tried it again since then.

John was an award-winning TV news producer. He covered many war zones for over 60 years, 78 countries and 35 war zones. The job, from what he'd seen, took a toll, PTSD, or post-traumatic stress disorder. He lives in fear of the day that's to come. After 35 years of treatment, there is no improvement.

In an actual application on a patient who had only months to live with terminal cancer, the nurse hands him the needle with a plunger on it, that he can push. She said, "Safe travels, my friend". He responded, "Goodbye my friend. I love you guys."

In March 2023, slowly over half a year of this writing, Canada's MAiD law will include people with incurable mental disorders. Actually, one can argue that this is already in effect, since my friends, Matt, and also Adam, were not terminally ill, only compounded their physical ailments with psychological problems.

Doctors like Ellen Wiebe, a Vancouver physician, will be able to help patients like John Scully. She's helped over 400 patients with physical incurable illnesses die with medical assistance. She believes that MAiD should be expanded to the mentally ill as well if there is no cure.

"As Canadians we have rights. Mental illness and physical illness can cause unbearable suffering and it's up to the person themselves to decide if they want to have assistance to die."

*****

Almost 2,000,000 people in Canada suffer from mental illness. That is a huge number of mentally ill people who could rush to the assistance of MAiD. Many of them are young people! One woman said, "MAiD was better than jumping off a balcony. If I can't say, enough is enough, then we are not living in a democracy."

Another man, interviewed by Avis Favaro, said he wanted to die since he was 11 years old. He's tried every kind of medication. He commented, "Everyone should be able to access this. There are so many people on disabilities that have been ignored for so long, there's going to be a rush for the doors."

Avis Favaro is a CTV news medical correspondent who specializes in health stories that make a difference in the lives of Canadians. The question is, "Can better treatments convince patients to keep going?" Dr. Wiebe, a champion for MAiD, observed that she'd like to see better health treatment in this country. No doubt about that.

Yet, there are health workers who are afraid in which direction the county is going. Dr. John Mahar: "We are having to fight with other doctors, not to kill our patients that we know could get better." He added, "it is state sanctioned suicide." He said that his profession tries to give hope. He said that he has a patient who told him, "I would not kill myself on my own, but I would kill myself through MAiD because that's not suicide." Also, in a 19-point report, one of which suggested that the procedure could not go ahead during a period of crisis for the patient, which is supposed to be "a failsafe", there is a way to get around that. A patient commented that a patient can lie about their state of mind.

Serena Bains is struggling with a life-threatening "pulmonary embolism", a condition that the medical profession did not take seriously. Her moods also swing go up and down. She's been on waiting lists with specialists for several years. She's also had to go without her medical drugs because she can't afford them. She rations her meds.

The recent report told Ottawa that a patient should get the full services of counseling and meds before they get MAiD. But that does not happen within Canada's clogged system with huge waiting lists! Avis Favaro commented, the system will allow you "to check out before you can get the services." Serena Bains said that currently the system protects her against herself. She really doesn't want to die, but if the mentally ill are included in the mandate, then when she is in at a low, she does not know what she will do.

41
One in Three
Not Good!

Dr. Mahar said that only one in three people in Canada have access to the mental healthcare they need. He further pointed out that only one in five children get the help they need, which is a "horrific reality".

Dr. Mahar is shocked that patients cannot get access to services they need. He went on to say, "If that isn't something that worries people, I don't know what to say about our Canadian society that we are offering death to people where treatment is available where you can't say to people who will get better and who won't." In a poll, 61% of Canadians agreed that MAiD should not be offered to people who are waiting for other treatment that might help them. Dr. Mahar continued to say, "You who have voted for this law have not understood vulnerability and what It means for your doctor to offer you death over life."

The contentious issue is whether mental illness is really incurable. Scientists around the world cannot agree which patients will recover and which won't. This question is of course a difficult problem in Canada because many patients do not have help to treatments and meds that they need because of an underfunded system and one that is backed up by waiting lines. Dr. Mahar said, "I have people who have come to me, who get better after 5 years, after 10 years, after 15 years." He is a proponent of hope, if only the system would give help!

Dr. Scott Kim, a bioethicist, says that Canada is liberal in its approach, whereas rules are stricter in the Netherlands and in Belgium where euthanasia has been practiced for two decades. Dr. Kim likes Europe's approach because people who would choose euthanasia would not be eligible if what they needed was better care. He observed that up to 70% of cases are rejected in the Netherlands because overwhelmingly there are other alternatives, which preserve life. Dr. Kim agrees with people who think euthanasia is okay, but they need to be alarmed in Canada, that there are not enough safeguards. So how do Canada's restrictions match with Europe's? Dr. Kim's assessment is that "the Canadian situation even at the legal level is much more permissive." When Avis Favoro said in her interview that Canada then would be the most liberal in the world in administering euthanasia for mental disorders, Dr. Kim commented, "without a doubt. No questions asked."

This liberal approach to making the mentally ill eligible for medical assistance in dying worries people like Serena Bains. Her approach is to build a strong support system with friends and family, a sort of buffer against the times when she feels low. Her work will also help at the disability foundation where she finds purpose as an activist in getting people with mental illnesses quicker help within the system. Serena is a champion of "consistent and accessible mental health services." She wants access to a psychiatrist and access to meds at no cost, or reasonable costs. "If you see us as disabled enough for medical assistance in dying, you should see us disabled enough to provide us with the accommodations and supports that we need."

But it seems that some people like John Scully see no other help, except that people like him put their hope in medical assistance in dying as a final way to end their suffering. His wife and family support him in his decision to end his suffering with dignity. For him, "there is no relief, so I have no alternative. I would have a dignified death with my family, probably play some music and I would die peacefully."

*****

I could see John Scully as eligible for MAiD because he is already 81 years old; he's had a full life and been a successful man. But with a young woman, like Serena Bains, the problem could simply be not getting counseling in a timely manner and the right meds at an affordable cost. It's disgraceful for this country that she has to ration her meds.

From what I've taken away in this W5 report is that the existing system is not fulfilling its mandate to give help to the sick in a timely manner. Words like access, waiting times, and proper meds and timely help from psychiatrics keep cropping up. If MAiD becomes accessible to the mentally ill within 9 months, three quarters of a year, then the "universal" healthcare system in Canada still has not become better. It will cover up, be a band aid for what is wrong with the system, that people are not getting the real help they need.

Just like an iceberg, 90% of the system is still underwater, dirty, and dangerous, untouched by air or sunlight. Our sickness remains hidden and unhealed, underfunded, and sluggish. The whole madness of wait times and crazy referrals remains uncured. We are like the boiling frog who is warmed in increments until the frog is boiled and dies! Look at the craziness in the United States with mass shootings, which have become part of the "norm". Utterly insane, but "accepted", even though not acceptable.

Well, we have 8 months to wait, for MAiD to make eligible those people seeking a way out of their pain because they are mentally ill and can't stand it anymore.

If there is a rush on the system, will we comply with the law of supply and demand by building MAiD centers all over the country, possibly next to hospitals, to process people who wanted to end it all. Will MAiD centers proliferate like gas stations? How do we reach the 90% of those sad people who are swamped under the iceberg who could have been helped if the system were right, if they could have been provided with the accommodation and the support they really need, so that they are given a real option in a well-funded, efficiently run, and humane medical system.

42
Personal Testimony

When I was a young man, still in my 30s, my first wife left me for a lawyer, a confident man with a golden tongue and great prospects. I was making minimum wages as a news reporter. I suppose I can't blame circumstances for her finding someone more right for her. Things, I suppose, went the way they were meant to be.

I was so depressed that I told my family back in Ontario I thought about committing suicide. They sent my younger brother to Grande Prairie, Alberta, which helped. He forged a future there for himself by becoming an electrician. I went into teaching, doubling my salary, but was completely unhappy and not suited to the job. I had a nervous breakdown. My doctor described it as post-traumatic stress disorder.

In the 1980s, it did not take long to get a psychiatrist's help. The healthcare system was not so broken then. I also had religious friends who spent a lot of time talking to me about the value of life and the possibility of finding a different direction. I found a lot of help, as well, from audio lectures done by an Australian psychiatrist, Doctor Claire Weekes, and her excellent book, Hope and Help for Your Nerves. She explained how the mind can go in circles, continually being sensitized by stimuli which you need to change. With the medication of Imipramine, counseling, and the help of a church, I slowly recovered. It took 3 years, a difficult journey.

Yet, if MAiD were around, I might have fallen through the cracks and actually ended my life legally. I had been hospitalized during my depression. Since my recovery, I got married and wrote some 30 books, available on Kindle and Amazon. I am 77 years old now, still feeling useful and productive by writing this book.

I think of John Scully and his situation at the age of 81. I know he tried suicide twice and has had decades of struggle with mental illness. Yet, at the end of W5, I wondered if his life could have been made bearable and still fruitful if we had a better system.

At the end of W5, the man is pictured walking on a wooded trail with his wife. "How's the river today?" "It was down and muddy, wasn't it?" "Looks clearer than before."

One wonders whether there is nothing left for John Scully, nothing to talk about, nothing to share. If only the system could take care of his pain through proper meds and a counselor with insight, he might still have some quality of life. Perhaps, there would be less demand for MAiD and more reaching down to the 90% drowning under the iceberg of insufficient funds and insufficient manpower to bring them up into the air and into the sunlight!

As for my own thoughts on the broken Canadian Healthcare system, the way it is, I do not trust it. I do not trust it when my wife is sick, and I need to call an ambulance. I do not trust it when I need a specialist's appointment and I have to wait a year to get it.

How did Canada get this way when European countries like Finland, the Netherlands and Belgium are faring way better, taking care of their citizens?

To have MAiD increase its parameters to the mentally ill, the frustrated and who knows, the disabled poor next who cannot afford care, is no answer. That is killing them and burying the problem! To me, that is barbaric and shameful for our country, the politicians and the powerful people are elected to make laws which fail to take care of the sick, the poor, the old and the dying.

My wife and I love two Canadian produced TV shows: Saving Hope and Transplant. These hospital shows depict doctors as caring for bloody patients coming into the ER from an accident, or patients coming in for cancer surgery.

However, so far, I've seen no theme on the waiting times in our society and the operations that are always, it seems, cancelled, or rescheduled like airplane flights. Nobody complains about untimely care on these popular TV shows, as if the problem of wait-times and a broken system do not exist. But then, like in the old days, doctors must live up to the caring and healing image of Dr. Ben Casey and Dr. Kildare. My wife and I love the new series, Saving Hope, where doctors are always looking out for the welfare of their patients despite the cost cutting necessities that the CEOs in the bureaucracy are faced with. I still pray that doctors are still good guys, maybe caught in a system that they themselves can't help. But who will fix it?

What a sad system we have now, when that great pioneer Tommy Douglas had such great hope for a universal healthcare system which could care for the country's own citizens, and which was such a humane example for the rest of the world!

43
My Classmate, Jim Moyer
Thoughts on His Obituary 2018

I knew Jim Moyer from grade 4 on at St. Joseph Elementary School in Kitchener. As a refugee I was put back two grades to learn English. Maybe, it was the malnutrition in the barracks in Austria. I was small for my age, and so moving from Sacred Heart School to St. Joseph School, I simply stayed in the same class they put me in. No moving ahead.

Jim must have been put ahead a year because he was so smart. Therefore, he was 3 years younger than I, which always made me feel self-conscious and embarrassed when somebody asked our age. I was older than any other kids in the class!

In grade 8, I had a 90% average. Jim had 91%. That 1% irked me, I suppose, because I had to work hard to get my grade. Jim had a photographic memory and just seemed to breeze through his high marks.

We never were really good friends, just classmates. He invited me over to his house one time in grade 8 to show off a motorized miniature snowmobile he'd built. The thing was driven by a Thimble Drome gas engine, and when Jim started it, it being winter, it skimmed across the snow like a rocket.

Jim was good with his hands. We had a wooden shelf project, which looked like a sailboat, to do in grade 7 Shop. Jim's boat looked finely sanded and shellacked; mine was a bit chunkier.

I won a $50 scholarship in grade 8, presented to me by Mayor Meinzinger. I think the Principal, Sister Gemma, named me for the award, instead of Jim, because I had been volunteering as a crossing guard and did other citizenship things around the school. She announced the highest marks to the class and said that there was only a hair's breadth's difference between Jim and me.

After Mayor Meinzinger presented me with the award, he delivered a lovely speech, sat down beside Monsignor Haller, turned purple, leaned against the Monsignor's shoulder, and died of a massive heart-attack. I witnessed that event which was scary. My father and several others carried the mayor outdoors into the fresh air, but that did no good.

Jim Moyer and I ended up in grade 9A at St. Jerome's High School. Grades were streamed from A to F in those days at St. Jerome's High School. It seemed that Jim's grades kept getting stronger by grade 10, while my grades weakened after grade 10.

I still squeaked my name into the honor roll for having a 76% average. Mom and dad were embroiled in heated arguments at the time, but I can't blame my declining grades on that alone. Jim plainly was smarter. He scored over 80%.

I remember Mr. McKay's grade 10 Math exam. I was still stuck on question #1, while Jim, as I glanced over, was already starting question #3. Incidentally, it was Mr. McKay's math class which was interrupted by the announcement that President John F. Kennedy had been shot to death in Dallas in a motorcade. My mother cherished his photo on the wall in our basement, along with a picture of the Pope and one of Jesus.

Only two other students seemed to stand out with increasingly better marks than Jim: Rick Moxon and Frank Meyer. Rick, I believe, went on to become a plastic surgeon. Frank Meyer went into Civil Engineering, along with Jim, eventually getting a Ph.D. An engineer friend told me that Jim and Frank were the two "brains" in the engineering department.

Anyway, by grade 11 Physics, I was getting average marks while Jim kept excelling. I remember switching to a light blue ink pen, like Jim used, to see if my marks would improve. It's silly, I know. When that did not work, I switched my slanted cursive handwriting to upright, thinking that teachers might notice my fresh new start. Superstitious habits did not work!

In grade 12, I had 55% in Math. I don't know what Jim, Frank or Rick got. Grade 12 was a traumatic year. I often suffered from migraine headaches and mom and dad continued to argue terribly, often escalating to violence.

Grade 12 was the deciding year for students who would go either into sciences or into arts at university. Jim had excelled and superseded my performance. He never raised his hand in class. Didn't need to, I suppose. Maybe, that's the assurance he had in his own ability.

I'm sure that Jim never gave me a passing thought in those high school days where our paths diverged. I've thought of him often over the years and suppose have been secretly envious of his success.

Math and Sciences simply eluded me. I had more of an inclination toward the Arts. That made all the difference in the world, as I took jobs as a news reporter and later as a teacher, experiencing tough trials and tribulations in that job market, which resulted in two nervous breakdowns.

During the Pierre Elliot Trudeau years, money and bursaries were plenty for lower middle-class kids like me to become a lawyer, doctor, or engineer. The door was open!

Dad, as a forklift driver on construction, would have been proud of me. Yet, I was poor in math, and was sucked into the hippie mentality of entitlement. There was no need to think about the future and the job market. I got distracted by the easy life of a university arts student. A degree in coffee shop was more in my line!

Jim breezed through his math and sciences in high-school and went straight into Civil Engineering. His co-ops paid for his university. That was smart! I continued with my summer jobs as a laborer on construction. I came out after a 4-year Double Honors in English and History with a $7,000 student debt. I carried that debt on through an M.A. year at McMaster University in 1972, coming out of that year with no prospect of a solid job, except maybe to continue on at Teacher's College.

Jim had his diploma in Civil Engineering in 1972. He had a solid job with Taylor Construction. He got married and refined his skills in the building trade as an architect and general contractor, let alone civil engineer. The Cambridge/Kitchener/Waterloo area offered him job contracts.

I was not happy in my M.A. year, making unwise choices in my electives: Restoration English, Milton's Paradise Lost and Chaucer. I would have done better with Mark Twain and John Steinbeck...but that is all hindsight.

My marks were strangely disparate:

- A First in Restoration English, which surprised me, the prof saying that my work was creative.

- A Second in Milton, satisfactory in comparing Milton's epic poem, Paradise Lost, with his book on the Art of Logic. This also surprised me because I hated Milton's pedantic poetry after I got into it.
- A Third or basically failure in Chaucer. "Hartig's work was poor. He is not recommended for a Ph.D." Originally, I loved Chaucer but experiencing the course under this prof at MacMaster, I hated the course, and I hated Chaucer.

I suppose I could have realigned my sights with a reapplication to an M.A. in History or possibly taken my master's over again at another university, but I saw a blank wall, namely Chaucer, blocking the way to higher aspirations in my academic career.

I moved back home and applied for unemployment money, for which my Teaching Assistantship entitled me, enough money for gas and Tim Horton's coffee where I sat reading War and Peace and Crime and Punishment.

Shortly after, I bought a motorcycle, a 350 cc Suzuki, two stroke, and moved out of the house into an abode full of hippies, the James Gang, on James Street in Waterloo. It was one of those no-exit streets off King.

I held a string of no-account jobs, earning no-account wages. I pumped gas, worked at Schneider's Meats, and became a common construction laborer to help pay off my student loan.

Jim could have been my boss, having achieved a higher social status as an engineer, architect, and general contractor. While I was a hippie, Jim eventually became a partner at Taylor Construction and eventually bought them out. He achieved success.

Jim loved boating. With houses and other big building projects, he must have made quite a good living. But he seemed to stay put around the Kitchener-Waterloo area all his life. I bounced around through several provinces from 1976 to 1986. I begrudged an education which seemed to corner me into a few possibilities which I did resented, like low-paid   news   reporter   or   stressed-out   teacher.

There are times when all the world's asleep
The questions run too deep
For such a simple man
Won't you please, please tell me what we've learned?
I know it sounds absurd
Please tell me who I am
Who I am?
Supertramp

44
Off the Beaten Path
Wrong Turn

This year, I almost died. I had an incident in September 2023. My heart rate jumped to 190 beats per minute. The ambulance took me to West Lincoln and they in turn drove me to Hamilton General because they did not have the qualified people to deal with my unruly heart. Within the week, an ICD or implantable cardioverter-defibrillator had been inserted into the left part of my chest. The ICD delivers an electric shock to restore a regular heartbeat when needed.

When I got home, I googled two of my old classmates, guys I'd been in class with from 9A to 12A, whom I found out had sadly passed away of cancer.

Frank Meyer was only 65 when he died of cancer on November 16, 2013. He had a successful asphalt company across Canada. Of course, he didn't use MAiD because medical assistance in dying had not been legalized yet, until 2016.

My other friend, Jim Moyer, died of cancer on Sept. 2, 2018. He, likewise, owned a successful construction business, being a respected general contractor, architect, and civil engineer. By then, MAiD had been legalized for two years. I do not know if he ever thought of medical assistance in dying, or if cancer meds kept his pains under control.

I was prompted to write a revised version of this book about MAiD since I'd already known two other friends who used the service. There were extra thoughts I wanted to add in a revision of my book.

However, my energy level was usually Zero during the day after my heart incident, and I was distracted with the daily News, the wars still brewing in Ukraine and now on October 7, 2023, the new war between Hamas and Israel. I remember our history classes when I was a boy and how the First World War broke out in the Balkan Powder Keg. Have we not learned anything?

Maybe, my revision won't matter if somebody pushes the red button on a few H-bombs. Anyway, memories started rushing back from the times of wasted years. I had to digress off topic as thoughts raced by, away from MAiD, medical assistance in dying, and simply dump thoughts as they rushed in, into this chapter of my book, because there was no other place, I could put them.

*****

I already had my 350 Suzuki motorbike. It was a good thing it was September, still good enough weather for biking. I already moved out of the house at home and paid my first and last month rent to the other three university students living in the townhouse behind St. Mary's Hospital. Mel and Bob were taking agricultural courses at Guelph. Karen was taking English at the University of Waterloo. They didn't mind a non-student who was working on construction to pay off his student loans. When I knocked at the door, with the ad in hand, looking for a fourth person to share rent, I remember Karen ogling me and drooping her ample breast over the arm of the chesterfield. She looked what experienced young men might call, "easy". I fit in quite nicely with this living arrangement. Bob and Karen later hooked up as an item.

A month into my new location, my dad knocked on the door. He didn't want to come in. We sat in his car while it started raining. He was ready to get an apartment and simply walk out on my mother. My sister had married by then and my brother was on the verge of flying out of the house on his own. Dad wanted me to get an apartment with him; maybe he lacked the courage to strike out on his own. I knew what that felt like. I said No. I felt that us as a duo would bring so many unhappy memories of arguments back that our association would be toxic for both of us. Dad would have to do the move on his own. I went back into the apartment. He drove off, maybe back home, maybe to the bed in the cellar of the house. Maybe mom and dad had made some "arrangement".

I was good for rent until November and then I moved out of the townhouse, not leaving a forwarding address behind. In the meantime, I'd been working on construction, saving money to pay for my student loan.

I knocked on the door of a house at the end of a little street, James Street in Waterloo. They were all University of Waterloo students, and they were receptive to someone with a motorbike moving in with them. I got the room next to the kitchen. I slept on a 4-inch foam mattress. All I had with me was a duffel bag of clothes and my violin case. I put off buying a car as long as I could.

Bruce ran the place. He looked like a pimply Buddy Holly with black horn-rimmed glasses, but his taste for music ran along the line of Gord Lightfoot. He'd strum up Every Highway at any time of day or night. You had to put up with it. I refrained from jamming along with my violin. Bruce lived upstairs in a little side room, off the bathroom. He had a wide-eyed girlfriend who looked like the Cheshire cat from Alice in Wonderland. She was wont to run almost naked with her panties into Bruce's room if anybody came upstairs. It was something we all got used to.

Mike was an M.A. student in English Literature snagging another room off the kitchen on the opposite end. He was arrogant and dirty-mouthed. I thought, "And he's an English student?" His girlfriend took the train in from Montreal at the end of each month. I wondered if I should have tried my luck doing an M.A. at the University of Waterloo. But then, that was the Road Not Taken.

A skinny long-haired student, Alan, was in engineering. He liked to build huge speakers which he'd sell for extra money. One speaker, which shook the house, actually blocked the doorway to his room because the thing stood 4 feet by 7 feet tall. The bigger the better!

Downstairs lived Mary who was finishing off her degree as a City Planner. She'd just broken up with her boyfriend. Because they were still on friendly terms, he carried her huge TV set into the house and on downstairs with herculean strength. They'd both been enrolled in brown belts in Tai Kwon Do.

I ended up doing most of the dishes each week because I could not stand it when they piled up at night with the person who was supposed to do them, ignoring his job. By the way, it was difficult getting up at 6 in the morning for construction work when the gang smoked their hash at night and told stories guzzling beer 'til the wee hours. But in those days, that was the lifestyle.

I remember a most notable supper of soup. It was rudely interrupted by grunting and groaning from upstairs, and then some obvious shaking of the ceiling. I wondered how much the mattress upstairs could take. Thank God, it subsided. I remarked, "Well, that was invigorating!" Some of us laughed.

I don't know what I was thinking. I let days drift by, thinking that I had enough youth to burn in my mid-twenties, that nothing in the future mattered. I hooked up with Mary downstairs and rarely came up for air.

Commitment was not on my mind. Deep-down I was seething with anger about the choices I made, about having to go to a laborer's job at six in the morning, about a slob like Mike getting his M.A. and probably his Ph.D. next year, about my dead-end future.

Mary had always wanted to work in British Columbia. She applied for a job there as a regional planner and got it in Chilliwack. I applied to Teacher's College at U.B.C. and was accepted, not seeing anything better to do. We lived together on the top floor of an old farmhouse. There were no jobs available for teachers. I finally got a job as a reporter at the Chilliwack Progress newspaper. My pay was half of Mary's. I sold my motorbike and puttered around town in a 1963 Volkswagen Beetle doing interviews for my stories. All this, while my friends, like Jim Moyer and Frank Meyer, were firmly grounded in engineering jobs, building well-paid careers.

Mary asked me one day if her co-worker at the regional office could move into the vacant apartment downstairs. I foolishly said, yes. Soon, she told me that she and he were in love and had an affair. It was time for me to move on. Any other guy would have clocked her new amour and rightly so, but my mind was in such a muddle, I simply didn't react that way. So many unsatisfied things were seething inside of me anyway. Lots of anger about pay, not getting ahead and the obvious double-cross by Mary and her boyfriend.

It was a good thing I'd sold my motorbike. I packed up my violin, some clothes and drove across the mountains, headed to Grande Prairie, Alberta. I'd read that there was a job available with another rag-tag newspaper, The Booster. I phoned the paper just to make sure. Yep, the job was still available, hoping to fill it by the end of the month.

I drove into 100 Mile House, somewhere in the mountains. The Super 8 seemed like a decent pit-stop. I couldn't sleep. I stared at the ceiling most of the night. I phoned a suicide hotline. The person at the other end was at least willing to listen to me. I felt bad, unlucky in love. On the way to 100 Mile House, I almost drove off a cliff on an impulse, but then, I didn't want to get my violin scratched in case Grande Prairie had an amateur orchestra.

Talking all night did me good. I had home fries and eggs before I left in the morning, before tackling my next leg of the journey to Alberta. I thought of Ian Tyson's song, Four Strong Winds.

The publisher of The Booster welcomed me warmly and showed me around the establishment which had its presses whirring and its darkroom redolent of chemical smells. "We're a small weekly but a proud paper that does good reporting." The editor took me for a beer at a local pub. He drank ginger-ale and confessed that he was a recovering alcoholic. I would start work the next day.

I rented a trailer that same day in a trailer court. "You can always sublet to help with the rent," said the manager. It looked like I had set roots in a new place, and it did not seem so bad. I tried to forget Mary and her new boyfriend and sunk myself deeply into work.

The Booster was a surprise to me. I loved the new job and shortly became its editor. Jack, the former editor, simply could not remain sober. The publisher asked me, "Are you able to handle the job as editor?" "Yes," I said. We talked about a thousand dollar raise in pay.

When I did not get a raise the next year, I quit and was hired as a high-school teacher at Crooked Creek. I doubled my salary but faced high stress in trying to get the kids to listen in my class. I had a nervous breakdown and looked to God for emotional support. I attended a Mennonite church in Grande Prairie and felt comfortable there. My nerves settled down. I bought a house and the rent from two roommates helped me with the mortgage.

My future wife, Marjorie, came into the picture about this time. She prefers to remain anonymous in all my writings. She moved to Grande Prairie from Ontario, specifically into the Mennonite community, to teach grades 6 to 8. We went for long walks together.

I sold the house and used the money to enroll in Canadian Mennonite Bible College [CMBC] in Winnipeg. I wanted "to find God" and I figured a religious institution which trained people as pastors would be the perfect place to find answers. It was also a safe environment because I enjoyed being a student and not a teacher.

My wife and I wrote long letters back and forth between Grande Prairie and Winnipeg. We got married in 1986. I switched my religious studies to French Literature through an agreement between CMBC and the University of Winnipeg.

I signed up for an exchange program with the University of Perpignan in southern France. I had just enough money from the sale of my house in Grande Prairie to fund my wife and myself for a year of living in France. After some foreign visa haggling, Marjorie was counted as the 20th "student" who would come to France with the "student group". Four of the group succumbed to culture shock and came back to Canada mid-term. Through some finagling by the Prof, Marjorie and I found a lovely granny suite in a home on Nungesser Boulevard. We had a lovely abode from the backyard of which we could see snow covered "Mont Canigou". The university was only a 10-minute walk away.

This digression should be enough to highlight the huge difference between Jim Moyer's career and my scattered experiences. I see a direct connection to the movie, The Humanity Bureau, starring Nicolas Cage, where people are given a "productivity score" in society, so that if they get assessed too low, they are sent to New Eden where, unknown to anybody, they are exterminated.

I wondered what such an agency would have done with me when I was in my mid-twenties, wasting my time in pubs at night, working at odd jobs below my education level and living like a hippie. The Bureau could have cleared out a whole nest of us hippies on James Street...but then, the Bureau would not have known that some of us made good later in life.

The mandate for MAiD next year on March 17, 2024, must be regulated responsibly, because it will expand to include the mentally ill, not just the terminally ill. How far will the mandate for MAiD keep expanding? Will the government make judgements about people who do not "produce" in society in terms of jobs, their abilities and handicaps?

I guess my unsettled job experiences have given me material for writing novels. However, I have not become a great, nor financially, successful writer. Our different stories, between Jim and me, remind me of Robert Frost's old poem about diverging roads. I'm still not sure whether my fork in the road was a blessing to learn more about human nature for my storytelling, or if my lifestyle in my mid-twenties was simply a curse of poor choices.

45
Choices and Destinies

Jim Moyer was 69 when he died in 2018 of cancer. Initially, when I found out through Google that he had died, I had a shameful thought: "Ha, I outlived him!" And then I checked myself. I would not wish cancer on anybody.

I, myself, have had chronic leukemia but my doctor says, if there's ever any cancer you want, it's leukemia; it can go for decades without ever breaking out. I'll probably die of congestive heart failure anyway since I have arrythmia and a weak heart.

I have two heart operations to my credit, one to get an artificial aortic valve, a St. Jude's, size 23, done in 1987, and one to fix an aortic aneurysm in 2017. As refugees, living in barracks, my family experienced poor conditions in war-torn Austria in the 1950s. I had tuberculosis and rheumatic fever as a kid, hence the bad heart.

I do not know if Jim would have chosen MAiD if his suffering got unbearable after he found out he had cancer. MAiD was already legalized in 2016 in Canada two years before he died. I would use the service only if I ended up brain dead or drooling with Dementia in a wheelchair. I'd make sure I included such a codicil in a living will. I'd also consider MAiD, if I had terminal cancer.

Things have changed so much in our society. As time goes by, more and more of my classmates are dying off. That is what mankind is heir to. I suppose I could have saved myself from two nervous breakdowns in teaching, had Jim and I still been equal in marks throughout high school and university. I might have gone into engineering myself.

I notice that people respect doctors and engineers more, even lawyers. But only a few people seem to be blessed with photographic memories, intelligence, health, a ripe old age, and a job they love...and while I think of it, a happy marriage too.

I missed the mark in several of these categories. Perhaps, that's what a heaven, or what other multiverses, are for...to realize your dreams in parallel universes. Perhaps I'd be Professor John Hartig in one of those other multiverses? Jim did not have two nervous breakdowns, like I did, teaching kids who did not want to learn. That was not his destiny. His destiny was a successful engineering career and a marriage that lasted 46 years until he died.

Jim seemed to be equal to the stress his job demanded as an engineer, architect, and general contractor. I look at his success with envy. I suppose if one looked at the human race as an actual race, Jim would have won. He had a boat, a lovely house and loads of money in the bank. My writings and my books get me very little money. However, such speculation, about what should have been, could have been and might have been, is wasted energy!

Sad that Jim had cancer and only lived to 69 years of age. If I were him, I might have chosen to use MAiD to end my life and go out in a painless death. I hope his meds and his treatment dulled his pain enough in that last year of his life in 2018 to give him some quality of life still able to enjoy the company of his wife and family.

I know from another friend, Matt Scholtz, that cancer is an insidious disease. Matt decided to check out by medical assistance in dying in 2023.

MAiD was not available when my former brother-in-law, Ken Janzen, who died of lung cancer in 2008 at the age of 37. My wife says he would never have chosen doctor assisted suicide.

In March 2021, MAiD permitted additional situations to use its service. People with disabilities and chronic diseases who are "in an advanced state of irreversible decline" and have "Intolerable physical and psychological suffering that cannot be alleviated under conditions the person considers acceptable."

The September 22, 2023, edition of the Canadian Mennonite noted that 31,000 Canadians died with MAiD between 2016 and 2021. Once the mandate expands to include the mentally ill in March 2024, the people who use MAiD are expected to use the service exponentially. This does not sit right with some religious affiliations like the Evangelical Fellowship of Canada [EFC] who have consistently opposed the legalization of assisted suicide.

EFC's director, Julia Beazley, cautioned that new mandates must not be seen as the solution to suffering and despair. Instead, the government should be looking to fund the meds and programs needed to keep people alive who are in dire need of other ways to keep them alive with a reasonable quality of life. The obvious roadblock is that there are not enough money, so it's the lack of money that forces people with sicknesses into a box from which they see no other way out. One activist against MAiD said, "assistance should include care that doesn't involve actively ending someone's life."

An eye opener for Canadians should be the fact that Palliative Care is <u>NOT</u> a right in the Canada Health Act.

According to Rhonda Wiebe, a Winnipeg resident, she believes that Canada has no business offering MAiD, until Palliative Care is a right for every Canadian. As it is, MAiD is becoming the go-to solution...and why? Often because of the lack of funds for other types of care which probably could work if made available.

My father-in-law, Wally, who is 94 finally got palliative care now, after the family physician stepped in. It's unfortunate that this need happened at the same time that my own heart jumped from 190 beats a minute to 30, nearly killing me.

We both have the same problem now, congestive heart failure. I have an ICD implanted in my chest which needs tweaking in the next two weeks. I asked the doctor what it would feel like if the defibrillator kicked in. "Like the kick of a horse," he said. He was not kidding, "but it would revive you enough to get you to a hospital." Happy news!

These days, while he has palliative care nurses coming to the house, is like a vigil. Some days he looks like he's ready to go; some days he rallies.

Anyway, my wife just got back this evening from her visit to dad's. This gives Wally's wife a chance to go out briefly for grocery shopping. The home-care nurses are not always available, so it's not a reliable service. At least, it is something.

The nurse said that a time will come when Wally has to be admitted to hospice care and be taken out of his beloved home, and that will mean the end of his life. It's been expected.

It's quite a production to get Wally onto his walker and then onto his commode. He's been having bouts of diarrhea and vomiting. I know what that's like. This is what we are facing now at the time of this writing, the final chapters of my book on MAiD, The Final Exit.

It's a struggle currently saying what I have to say because of my own heart failure. I have Zero energy and hopefully, the next cardiologist's visit in Hamilton will give me answers about what to do to give me more quality of life. The publication of this book will come before either of our stories, either my father-in-law's, or mine, will play out.

Sometimes I feel like it's a race now, between dad and myself, who will go first. Of course, he's 94 whereas I have recovered enough to be able to make additions to my book. I also spent all afternoon making photocards out of some of my best prints, mainly sunsets, flowers and morning star mill photos. I thought maybe the church might use them as a fundraiser.

Shame that the images are saved on my external hard drive on my computer. If I go first, then nobody would know what's on my computer, valuable copies of my books and also pictures I've taken over the years, but who will know? Or care?

I wonder if dad knows that if he is moved to hospice care, then that's it! It will be the place where he'll die. Removing him from his beloved home would be so traumatic! Would he rage, would he be suppliant because he is too old and sick to rage? Nothing at all like Dylan Thomas wrote about in his poem, "Do not go gentle into that good night, to rage against the dying of the light!"

John 21:18 [18] Truly, truly, I say to you, when you were young, you used to dress yourself and walk wherever you wanted, but when you are old, you will stretch out your hands, and another will dress you and carry you where you do not want to go.

*****

I told my wife that I wanted the cheapest possible funeral. The local funeral home director lives in one of the richest houses in Vineland.

I don't even need a celebration of life. A small marker where I'm buried would do. I think MAiD is a sensible service in our society, though I hope that it is not misused for people who are mentally ill and simply are tired of living and want to end it all. Regulation has to be sensible!

I think there is an irony in the phrase, "the human race". The human race is intent on making achievements and jobs, in fact, all of life, into a race. It's like the one who has the most accumulations at the end of life is the winner!

People have an instinct to collect riches during their working years, so they have enough to last them through old age. Yet, there are so many stories of gifted people dying in poverty in their advanced years. During the race of life, one must be wise in one's investments.

Jim already won the race of careers and success by what he accomplished in his 69 years, as a Civil Engineer. How do I accept coming in second or even last, gracefully!

We strive and we thrive during our young years, so that we can enjoy "the golden years". But if disease or dementia sneaks up on you, then perhaps MAiD could be a blessing...maybe a wise foresight to write MAiD into a living will while you still can.

*****

In the history of the Cosmos, we are nothing. As galaxies fly further away from us, the 1% difference in grade 8 and the divergent roads we took as old classmates between Jim Moyer and me do not matter to the fleeting stars. We are all of us dust in the wind.

Our planet Earth might not matter in another 5 billion years when our Sun expands to engulf Mercury and Venus, making it too hot to survive on Earth. We should have voyaged elsewhere in space by that time, and by that time, Jim nor I would be a second thought to the swirling actions of our universe. If there is a Heaven, we'd have other worldly values to follow; if there is no Heaven and no God, what's it all matter, this difference between Jim and me.

*****

Perhaps, advice to those of us who are not as successful in life, is that old adage to just do the best you can, with whatever you've been given. Don't sweat the fact that not everybody is born an Einstein.

THE ROAD TAKEN
By John Hartig
Dedicated to my wife, Marjorie,
Monday June 11, 2001

Something to find leads me away,
To woods and lonely trails unseen,
To question the road, I've taken...
And the different future
that might have been.

Some trail leads me,
to waterfalls that crash.
My eyes see sparkles,
in a single splash...
Tiny drops, like people,
that tumble and toss,
and teem and toil,
And run...oh, where?
Like love, like life, so precious,
Like things, not always fair!

I imagine a droplet is the sun,
A splash - the galaxy,
Our existence - a miracle,
Our universe - you and me!

Seeing is more than eyes alone,
And more than merely looking.
We have a mind, a heart, and soul,
To behold wonder within the whole.

46

Interview With
A Life Enrichment Aide

Private Interview:
Sept. 1ˢᵗ, 2023

There is a hidden irony in being a "Life Enrichment" Aide in long-term care, especially since MAiD was legalized in Canada in 2016.

One such Aide, whom I identify as neither male nor female, in fact "anonymous," expressed "their" objections about the current trend in Canada where MAiD is promoted. This individual felt that they had to say something, not being comfortable with the pressured, active way MAiD is promoted in Long-Term Care.

"It's not my way of thinking," they said in the interview. They felt like a gag order had been imposed on them, not to say anything about the ethics of MAiD to clients asking questions in the seniors' home. They felt that they'd be reprimanded for talking to clients about their personal beliefs and possibly lose their job.

Life Enrichment Aides are under the direction of the Life Enrichment Coordinator. They all fall under the authority of the DOC, or Director of Care, of the home. In turn, they are under the direction of federal law and the policies promoted by the federal and provincial governments.

As a worker, under other authorities, Life Enrichment Aides are responsible for planning activities, evaluating programs, communicating programs, and effectively facilitating them in the Long-Term Care Home. Aides are also responsible for assessing residents and establishing goals for them, depending upon their needs and abilities. Much of this is paperwork, involving progress notes, care plans and quarterly reviews.

Since MAiD has been offered in Long-Term Care Homes, Aides are faced with personal concerns about freedom of expression and beliefs and how much they can or cannot interact with clients about the recent, legalized introduction of medical assistance in dying, available to those who are suffering either from a terminal illness, or from incurable diseases. Clients have questions, and they are prone to ask people, which means the Aides, whom they trust and with whom they interact on a daily and personal bases, what their opinion is about MAiD. A client is not inclined to open up with the higher ups, the people in charge of the home, about such personal concerns.

The Life Enrichment Aide whom I interviewed believed that dying, even with medical assistance, is still suicide and that a person taking such a step would only be trading worldly suffering for an eternal suffering in hell. That individual was perplexed about how to compartmentalize her Faith, when medical assistance in dying was so actively promoted by the government in long-term homes. Therefore, no matter how good a Life Enrichment Aide was in caring for their clients, the ability to share personal things and honestly answer any questions about whether MAiD was "right or wrong" was discouraged by the administration. The Life Enrichment Aide must walk a fine line, and answer, "I don't know," or refer the client to a councillor or a CEO, higher up on the administrative hierarchy.

The Life Enrichment Aide is not comfortable with what our current practices are doing to future generations who will be educated that medical assistance in dying is simply what happens to seniors in an enlightened, advanced society.

MAiD would slowly be accepted as the natural way for seniors to end their lives. In March 2024, MAiD would also be made available for irremediably, mentally ill people.

Some religious groups and some health-care workers are concerned about the broadening eligibility for MAiD. Where will the inclusivity for MAiD stop?

"I don't like it," said the Aide. "I don't think dying with MAiD is necessarily dying gracefully." This professional suggested that MAiD is convincing people, in fact, to use it, from the subtle propaganda of language, like "dying with dignity" and embracing death, like "falling asleep."

"As for me," suggested the Aide, "I am not allowed to influence people in any way to change their mind." In fact, the Aide has to support a client's journey towards MAiD. "It's like when a person gets ill, the administration swoops in with the MAiD program." This tactic, said the Aide, is when a person is the most vulnerable. The process from the moment of application takes three months.

Alzheimers and Dementia patients who are in lock-down are most vulnerable. Often the family does not want to deal with a relative who is no longer "with it," a burden to the family and costing too much money to keep them living. The most cost-effective way to deal with such old people is to give them a way out, a painless death.

The Aide, whom I interviewed, acknowledged that the government was actively training staff in seniors' homes to accept MAiD. "They are training us in the program." The worry doesn't stop there. "If you do not agree with the policy, you get fired."

There are ramifications that come out of such a program. If the client is wealthy, then the family might hurry the death of that client to hasten the family's inheritance, and so the family puts pressure on the client to accept MAiD, as the best thing for the client and for the family.

Money, of course, is a moving factor behind the whole scene. Certainly, for the government and its expenses in sustaining the lives of old folks, and certainly, for the family, if they want to go on with their own lives and no longer be bothered with visits to their aged relative in the home. Mental and emotional pressure can be applied to the client whose energy and ability to fight back may not be there anymore.

According to the Life Enrichment Aide, people should be afraid for future generations who will accept MAiD as a good and natural practice for a modern society. The DOCs, Directors of Care, are already cautioning their staff on what to say and what not to say about MAiD, obviously favoring the program as an enlightened and merciful practice.

The Life Enrichment Aide, whom I interviewed, is worried about where the eligibility for MAiD will stop and also about the staff's freedom for personal chats with their clients. In the current situation, if they say something, they will get castigated or worse, get fired!

The question too is who is introducing the program, its policy, its ethics, and its safeguards? Legislation comes from above, but some people, who are on the lower rung of decision making, see the program expand and actively implemented in an uncomfortable direction.

*****

ADDENDUM:

Although a Christian, I do not believe in a God who would condemn you to eternal damnation if you chose MAiD to escape your pain.

At my age, I go to bed a lot to ease my daily aches and pains with arthritis. You go to bed thinking that a couple of hours in bed would take away your aches and pains, but when you get up, nothing has changed. Each day, you wake to the same thing. Everything hurts. Sleep, except an eternal sleep, does not take anything away.

I admit that I'd use medical assistance in dying, if I faced a terminal illness and if pills did not manage the pain. People choose MAiD to make the pain stop. They want a way out!

Senior pain could be managed, if only we did not have a broken health-care system. Waiting times and access to specialists are ridiculously stymied. It's shameful in a country like Canada, which is expanding eligibility for MAiD as a cost-effective means of ending people's lives, instead of taking care of them to prolong their lives with acceptable management.

What is a hurting senior supposed to do to make their pain stop? Saving money is the driving force behind the government's expansion of MAiD services, using such euphemistic language as dying with dignity and going to sleep. The campaign program for such, is attractive for those who are suffering day by day.

When I think of pain in old folks, I get angry, when the war in Ukraine and other hot spots in the world are wasting the limbs and lives of young bodies thrust into conflicts created by politicians with worldly ambitions. Reminds me of Napoleon on his white steed at Waterloo manoeuvring his troops like little tin soldiers to be cannon fodder for the British artillery.

Within the forces of history and the lives of healthy, young men and women, it's the weak and the poor who suffer. The aged especially who simply don't want to wake up anymore to their aches and pains every morning, where they suffer the same old thing, there must be relief!

Canada's broken health-care system cannot manage the care of its seniors. There is no way out, except for MAiD, the promise of ending chronic pain in the oblivion of an endless sleep. Yes, I would succumb to the use of MAiD and be thankful for such a service if there was no way out, if there was no acceptable, manageable quality of life. If our system were not broken, then the pressures of money and accessibility would not be there...but alas old age prolonged costs money!

The current state of affairs reminds me of the Nicolas Cage movie, "The Humanity Bureau," filmed in 2018, where people had to meet a "productivity quotient" or else get deported to New Eden, where secretly, they were euthanized.

The mercy in MAiD is a difficult question. Its eligibility could be a slippery slope to an "inhumanity bureau" for who lives and who dies. Is mercy killing moral? Surely, the act in some cases would be a thankful blessing.

What is a human life worth? Is prolonging life, under well-funded management, guaranteeing an acceptable quality of life, an acceptable thing? Do we have the money to take care of our suffering seniors?

Hitler had some such notions about state assisted dying. He applied the practice to races and ethnic groups; we apply the practice to old folks.

There are so many moral questions involved. Is it right to end a terminal illness? Is it right to end insufferable pain, to recognize the difference between the wealthy and the poor, to find "solutions" to societal ills, to weigh the value of people who are a benefit to society and those who drain society. Where does enlightenment bless our society, and where are we driven back to the dark ages? Where is our hope and where is our enlightenment?

Who legalized this conundrum we are faced with now? In short, the Trudeau government!

The Trudeau government legalized MAiD in June 2016 after the Supreme Court ruled that parts of the Criminal Code outlawing assisted suicide violated the Charter of Rights and Freedoms. The pressure to legalize MAiD came from forces below, from articulate sick people who saw no other means to end their suffering. So now, the terminally ill have a legal means to control their own deaths.

However, for the future, we must have safeguards, laws in place which will prevent the government, from exercising its powers from above, dictating to old folks who is no longer useful in society and who is too sick to keep alive because the government can't afford it.

Also, in terms of eligibility, laws must be in place to prevent people who simply want to die because they are tired of living, or people who are depressed and can't get help because of a glutted system.

Euthanasia is the inoffensive term used for a merciful death. Arguments persist whether it's a blessing or a curse, whether eligibility should be strictly limited or applied on a broader basis. Where are we headed? While we argue about the ethics of all this in the West, we have two huge wars in the East, the one between Israel and Hamas and the one between Ukraine and Putin. Huge waste of human lives. Huge damage to bodies whose parts could have been used in transplants to save others. God and his angels are thinking, "What are these humans thinking!"

I'm concerned because I am 77 years old and who knows what seniors' home my wife and I will end up in? Will we still be together or put into separate rooms or separate Long-Term Cares? Where are we all headed in the sunset of our years? Where is our strength to say something, as we are funnelled, channelled, and processed in a failing system of care.

47
Conclusion

What are the answers to life? To the universe? We have astrophysicists who have discovered black holes in space, new worlds which possibly could sustain life. Space travel within our solar system and beyond, all that is within our grasp. We cure new diseases, we prolong life, but eventually we all must accept our fate, for mankind must die. Time is an arrow that moves forward and ages us all towards our final exit.

Perhaps, all we can hope for is three square meals a day, a good job, leisure time with good hobbies and a satisfying partnership in a marriage. Four score years and ten with reasonable health and then dying in one's bed in peace.

I do not like the belief of one character in a kung fu movie, "Lady Dragon", 1992, because he saw the dark side in everything, He summed it all up this way, "Life is a bitch and then you die." There's got to be more to life than merely living!

As biological entities, we are prone to wear and tear, to sickness and cancers invading our bodies. We've come a long way in treating and curing things, but the inevitable must happen. We cannot control the arrow of time and the fact that we age and wear down.

Perhaps, the next stage of evolution is the consciousness of AI, Artificial Intelligence, and self-replicating robots. Perhaps, that will be a step to conquering mortality, but not with us. Self-replicating robots won't need MAiD, and of course, they can always get spare parts.

If there ever is a transition where human beings are replaced by thinking robots, then MAiD might usher in that new era by culling the herd, so to speak, by getting rid of the irremediably ill, disabled and the aged who are in chronic pain.

Perhaps, our role has served its purpose, and we are scheduled for extinction. This does not have to be if we are wise. With our intelligence, we have the capacity to manage climate change and even a transition to the next stage of evolution, even if it is self-aware robots. As to our individual mortality, we need to learn acceptance, and take our final exit with grace and courage. My boyhood friend, Matt, waved goodbye to his friends from the third-floor apartment, doors open to the pergola, knowing that those people would go on to deal with the little things in their lives. He would have to give up his consciousness, his connection to the world. The needle would have put all the lights out in his awareness, as he fell asleep into death, into possibly oblivion, or as he hoped, a pain free after-life with Jesus.

Somehow, I suspect that people who chose MAiD would have chosen it, if the only thing it gave them was oblivion, just to get rid of the pain. That's human, all understandable.

Meanwhile, the world would bumble along with its politics, wars, with progress towards new medications and inventions and discoveries in outer space. Without Matt, without Adam, without my brother-in-law, Kenny, and all the loved ones who now only exist in my memory.

Who knows if we will share the Earth with thinking machines? Or be taken over by them. It's an interesting future which we have before us on planet Earth.

Of course, it doesn't have to go in a negative direction, if we control our inventions and actually find a cure for cancer first, before we invent things like self-aware machines. Surely, while we have life and control over our biological destiny, we will find humane and better ways of dealing with death, for the aged and the sick, once our time on Earth is done.

*****

"There's got to be more to life than just living," Foyle said to the robot.

"Then find it for yourself, sir. Don't ask the world to stop moving because you have doubts."

"Why can't we all move forward together?"

"Because you're all different. You're not lemmings. Some must lead, and hope that the rest will follow."

"Who leads?"

"The men who must...driven men, compelled men."

"Freak men."

"You're all freaks, sir. But you always have been freaks. Life is a freak. That's its hope and glory."

"Thank you very much."

"My pleasure, sir."

"You've saved the day."

"Always a lovely day somewhere, sir," the robot beamed.
Then it fizzed, jangled, and collapsed."
— Alfred Bester, <u>The Stars My Destination.</u>

*****

Acceptance is the big virtue which we must cultivate, as
a society, to face our mortality with maturity and courage.
Maybe MAiD is a service which helps us in that direction,
after all.

The Welsh poet, Dylan Thomas, wanted to rage against
the dying of the light, but that is useless, because he was a
drunk and a cynical human being. In old age, a person is
feeble, sick, and unable to rage against death anyway.
Maybe our education system needs a course on dying, on
mortality and living with pain and about being satisfied
with a life well lived. Maybe there is a gracefulness in how
to die? Lucky are those who can also do it peacefully.

I Walked to Kenny's
Grave Today
I walked to Kenny's grave today...
Snowflakes fell down
Like little kisses from heaven.
Canada Geese honked far off,
In their flight to who knows where?
I shed a tear...

I couldn't locate the tree, Kenny,
Where your mom lay?
They all looked the same to me.

So many names along the way,
I touched the stones and brushed the snow.
Where are you, Kenny, where did you go?

I looked up as I went...
Snowflakes touched my face,
Like little kisses from Heaven sent.

A dog barked in the cold, cold, air.
A sad thought came...are you really there?
A truck changed gear on a nearby road...
Sound of a jet plane headed someplace
[warm I hope].
This death, this everything...so unfair!

These cemetery paths
Remind me of that old Beatles' song,
"The long and Winding Road"...
Which one will lead me to your door?

Snow-limned branches hung above my head;
Old knots and scarred bark with moss.
A black squirrel scampering
Nimbly from branch to branch;
My soul mourned your recent loss.

Ah, here you are, Kenneth Janzen: 1970-2008.
A plastic marker, no gravestone yet,
Same lane as Oma and Opa Boldt,
Just a couple of doors down,
Is it comforting that you are neighbours?
Or don't those things matter anymore?

Birds chirp cheerily, a lonely dog barks once more...

At what?
Is there any sense to me being here?
Making footprints in the snow,
In my fear...and anger?

No more NHL cups, Kenny,
No more Coffee Crisps or chocolate pudding
[To make those horrible meds go down]
I hope you're eating a big fat juicy steak right now!

My face turns upward toward the sky.
I feel an angel has brushed me by.
Snowflakes and kisses
Sent from Heaven above,
Touched my face with tender love.

-- *John Hartig (Friday Feb. 1, 2008)*

48
And yet,
Some After-Thoughts

We are the victims of a Natural Law and Natural Selection that we don't even understand. At 7 billion people on this planet, maybe Mother Nature is at work pruning its tree, cutting off the useless and dead branches and getting rid of the excess. Those who can live life to the fullest have always survived, until they themselves fall victim to old age, sickness, and the dying of the light. The people, once known as Eskimos [in a day when that term did not offend anybody], were known, for their own strict survival laws to put their aged or sick on an ice floe, to set them adrift in the cold Arctic water, so they would slowly fall asleep and perish, probably as nourishment for the fishes, to complete the great cycle of life and death.

There are two movies which stick in my mind, which I hope never to come into reality. Soylent Green, a 1973 film, starring Charlton Heston and Edward G. Robinson.

In an overpopulated future, people's food is supplemented by Soylent products. When they die, people are lulled to sleep with their favourite music and put on a conveyor belt to be processed into Soylent green protein tablets. Heston, the cop, finds out the truth: "It's people! Soylent Green is made out of people!" There you have a planet with too many people, hiding a dark secret for its survival.

The other film is The Humanity Bureau, a 2017 film, starring Nicolas Cage and Sarah Lind, about a futuristic America where climate change has turned the Midwest into a desert. A government agency called the Humanity Bureau is assigned to judge the "productivity quotient" of citizens. If they are not productive, they are designated to New Eden, which promises a better life, but is an extermination camp, thereby pruning the useless limbs within society.

Sunset Manor?
Short Story
By John Hartig

"Here comes the Gestapo!" said head nurse, Alice Smith. She hated these three-month inspections. More of their seniors were taken away each time, processed and treated through the government's medical help in dying.

Alice had been struggling with her own sense of right and wrong ever since she worked at Sunset Manor taking care of clients at the home. She hated the idea of taking seniors away from the home to be processed ever since the parameters for the service had expanded.

A decade ago, during Doug Ford's time and his "for-profit" seniors' homes in Ontario, and also, the Liberal policies under the Justin Trudeau government, the parameters for doctor assisted euthanasia had indeed expanded, first from the terminally ill, then to include the mentally ill, and finally to include seniors who simply said, "I've had enough of living. I want to go Home."

The Director of the home, John Hart, sat behind the desk in the boardroom. He had with him the chief accountant of the home, who sat behind a stack of papers. The home's lawyer was also present, as was the government's rep, Tim O'Reagan, who sat silently off to one side of the proceedings. The session was recorded. Four clients were called into the boardroom, one at a time.

"This is just a formality," said John Hart to the first of these clients, Nancy, who had been a resident of the home for 25 years.

"You've been with us a long time," said the Director. "We have tallied up what you owe us for the last month of stay and of food. It's all on paper here, a copy of which our accountant will pass on to the government's representative, Mr. O'Reagan. We also deducted the cost of the end-of-life procedure and your funeral cost. Anything left over, is to be appropriated by the government for incidental fees."

This meant that Nancy had nothing left in her bank account and certainly nothing left for any disbursement to relatives. After a signature, Nancy was escorted out to the foyer. She could see the van idling in the parking lot in front of Sunset Manor, as it did every three months. It was routine now. She was bright enough to picture being turned upside down and shaken for any loose change which might dislodge from her clothing. She would leave this world with nothing.

Tim O'Reagan leaned over to the Director next to him in the boardroom and whispered, "Make sure we have copies, as well, of the medical report for each client and consent form to go ahead with end-of-life." Armed with these reports, O'Reagan was assured that everything was in order, all the t's crossed and the I's dotted for these Sunset Manor clients who were now ready to leave the premises. The term "inmates" almost came to mind, but he dismissed that. This was not a prison.

The Director pretty well repeated the same speech to the other three clients who would board the van shortly.

He got their signatures. They were ushered out of the boardroom. This did not take long.

The large van, parked outside, had lots of room for 4 wizened old passengers. Sometimes, the van drove off with 6 or 8 people. This was the usual routine. Once clients were collected, it stopped briefly at Tim Horton's for a treat and then proceeded to the hospital wing, known for giving people, mostly seniors, their end-of-life "care."

Nancy was ready. The government rep, O'Reagan, checked off a box on his clipboard.

"Three months ago," he said, "you were not ready to come with us. How are you doing now?"

Nancy responded, "I've just celebrated my 93rd birthday. I ache all over. I can't see well, so the library down the street is useless to me. I also can't hear very well, so I cannot enjoy the classical music I love. I can't taste my food anymore...so I'm ready to go."

"You've made a good decision," said O'Reagan. He had several boxes to check off, which gave him a matrix, a list, called "Enjoyment of Life." The quotient was too low for Nancy to keep on living. He smiled at her, and a personal aid escorted her out the door. There wasn't anything to take along, except a picture of her son who never visited anymore.

"Are you sure it's painless?" she asked O'Reagan.

"It's like a lovely dream," assured the government rep. He had been taught what to say to these seniors who would soon leave life behind.

The process was indeed painless. The patient was put into a bed. The first medication was a sedative. Then the client was given a plunger, so that he or she could use their own thumb to press it, injecting the second medication into the bloodstream. A deep coma followed. The third medication was administered by the physician which stopped the person's heart. Music that the client had chosen would play softly in the background throughout the whole procedure.

O'Reagan did not go into all the details with Nancy, however. Better not to fret the poor old woman with details.

He said again, "Yes, it's like going into a lovely dream, a comfortable sleep."

"It will be wonderful not to wake up every morning to my aches and pains. I'm ready to go," she said.

Lydia was another matter. She was still a healthy 85-year-old. However, she was now indigent. Sunset Manor took the last of her money. $8,000 for the food and room covering this month's care. She was scheduled for a move to a less fancy and less caring home for the aged. Sunset Manor was "for-profit," and if you could pay, the home showed all the solicitude it could muster for its paying clients.

Instead of downsizing to a less-expensive home, Lydia chose to die. A move would be too much. "I'm tired of moving and of living," she confided to the director.

John Hart understood, but his hands were tied. He really cared about her, but once the client admitted that he or she had enough of living, he was obligated to record that and to pass the memo on to the government agency. He hugged Lydia and said, "I hope you enjoyed your stay with us. It's been a privilege knowing you. We will miss your piano playing in the lounge."

The other two clients were clear-cut cases. Lawrence who suffered from early onset dementia, a 65-year-old, who would never enjoy his retirement years. While still competent, he had signed a paper saying he wanted to use the government's offer to be processed into a painless death. He lined up at the door of Sunset Manor, ready to be escorted to the van.

Some seniors stood by and waved to him. He did not wave back. He stared at people with blank eyes that showed there was no Lawrence anymore behind them.

Michael was the last client ready to be escorted to the van. He'd had chemo and radiation for the cancer in his sinus cavity, but the side-effects of persistent pain and weight loss made him realize that the "cure" was worse than the disease. He hated the feeding tube he had to use. He wrote on a tablet, "My family doesn't need this. I'm ready to check out." He also could no longer talk because the tumor they took out froze his vocal cords.

Michael was 77 years old. He had been a successful writer, with 30 books to his credit. He had been a great "basso profundo" in his church choir. All that was gone now.

"I've had my life," he wrote on his tablet, "it's time to step aside."

The director, John Hart, nodded that he understood and hugged the man. Patted him on the back and handed him over to the aid who was loading clients onto the van. The van now had 4 new clients. It drove off to Tim Horton's for a brief coffee break. A donut too, a last treat before going to the pain-free processing center behind the hospital. Unfortunately, Michael could not participate in this last treat. He sat by, watched, and listened to idle conversation.

Arrangements had already been made for those who preferred cremation over the traditional burial. The government even offered "green burial." All paid for by the last of their money and of course, supplemented by government funds if necessary. The end-of-life service was very cost-effective overall, compared to what it would cost to keep these people alive.

All was good, they were being cared for, or taken care of if you prefer.

Tim O'Reagan had other senior homes to attend to, fulfilling his duties in a staggered schedule week after week. His van typically drove away with several to half a dozen clients per week, on a three-month rotation basis, visiting different homes, collecting seniors who were eligible for this pain-free service. He had heard one of the seniors joke recently, pointing to the van, "Here comes the Grim Reaper." He ignored the remark. He was only doing his job, and besides, the service was a mercy to those who were suffering.

Sometimes, he did not like his job. However, driving clients to a painless death was something he was convinced was good for them and for a progressively minded society. Someday, he himself would have to submit to the procedure.

He thought about his own old age. He sighed, and muttered, "Oh well."

49
Two Poems

When I write about a topic which moves me, I often write poetry, and so it is with MAiD which made me think of old age, of the passing of time, of endurance, and pleading.

There is no need to read these poems if that is not your thing. But if it is, then I hope you can identify with my emotions about our mortality. The following two poems come from two photos I took during a photo jaunt in the Niagara Region. "A Prayer from a Lonely Tree" and "The Gnarly Old Oak".

A Prayer from a Lonely Tree
by John Hartig
May 22, 2023

We are a Rare Earth Phenomenon, God aside,
Amid 2 billion galaxies, we are one of a kind.
There are 400 trillion suns in our Milky Way
2 billion rocky earth-like planets, they say.
7 billion humans thriving on this tiny blue dot,
which is incredibly right,
not too cold and not too hot.

The Fermi Paradox,
a thoughtful question asked,
"Where are the others?"
In all this black vast real estate,
Do we not have a mate?

The James Webb Telescope,
floating a million miles away,
searches for answers
which remain unanswered to this day.

We've discovered 5,000 exoplanets, they say,
where life may be or might have been.
Were those other worlds,
spared from original sin?
What does it all mean?
This searching, this seeking, this yearning,
Is there meaning in the universe?

Even if God does not exist,
Is there meaning?
Or are we an accident,
Leading futile lives
Of desperation?

There must be meaning,
because it is our very existence
that makes it so!
We are atoms that think, self-aware.
We search, we seek and yearn.
We ask in our inner core,
questions which are passed on,
to other curious minds
from ancient lore.

We give meaning to the stars,
to the universe and to life,
because we can ask
and wonder what we are.
The universe otherwise

has no meaning at all.
Who would know it is there?
And that we exist?

We are a miracle, so special,
so precious in the starry sky
that comes and goes,
like a silent sigh.
It's our mind that wonders,
about this unknown galaxy
about lightyear distances,
about time and space
We are graced with inspiration,
and aspiration, and the ability to ask,
so simple a question, as in days gone by:
"Twinkle, twinkle little star,
how I wonder what you are?"

Such a blessed thought,
and a humbling grasp of awe,
how our imagination can link
anthropomorphism to what we think,
to the simple meaning in a tree,
when its branches stretch out
in a seeming plea
to warn us to stop
our suicidal ways,
to become good stewards
of Mother Earth
for the rest of our days.

I saw such symbolism in my photo,
of a scraggly old pine tree
perched above a lonely rock,

looking like it was pleading,
please, please, please listen, oh humanity,
before it is too late
to save me,
to save you,
and to save this gift of meaning
that I send out in prayer
from this humble rock
to the silent stars above
as a humble message from my love...
before it is too late.

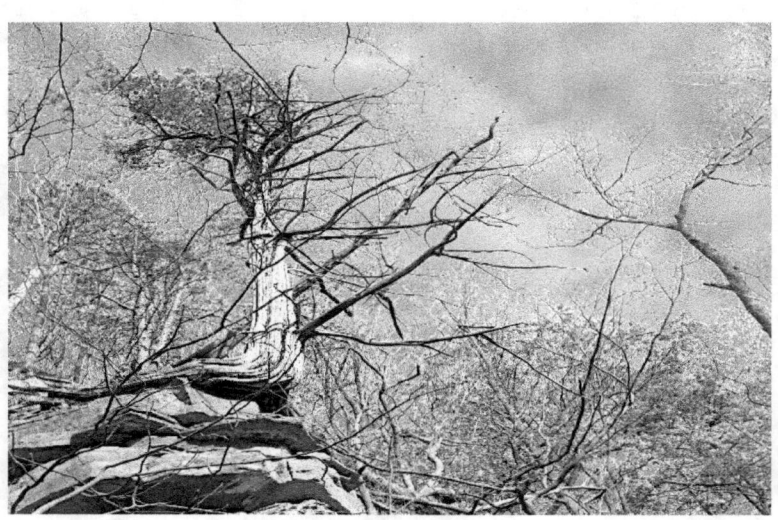

*****

The Gnarly Old Oak
by John Hartig
May 22, 2023

My camera lens is filled with the gnarly branches,
of the magnificent oak, standing tall and proud,
in its old age.
I snapped the photo to preserve the memory,
of the years and scars that wood endured.

What winds and climes this tree must have weathered?
Painful heat, heavy rains, and freezing snow.
If only its gnarly branches could tell the story,
how its skin got scarred, how it got old wounds,
signs of brave endurance.

There is a gnarly beauty in this ancient tree,
which stands high and proud,
in divine symmetry.
The knobbiness boasts of a quiet humility,
that has stood the test of time and of many years.

Gnarled and worn, the old oak tree stands resolute,
speaking to me of silent secrets that touch my soul,
a message of strength, endurance, and of pain
telling my old bones to endure the same.

I admire the old oak and its scarred wooden bark,
wondering if my frail body will likewise last through,
the test of time,
and bear up to tribulations,
like this brave old tree endured,

beyond the days of its prime.

Yes, I admire the wooden age of this old oak tree,
and wonder if my frail humanity,
will weather my own passing years?
Will I have the quality?
to endure my own deformity,
 as I grow old.
Will I be as strong and bold,
as this old oak tree?

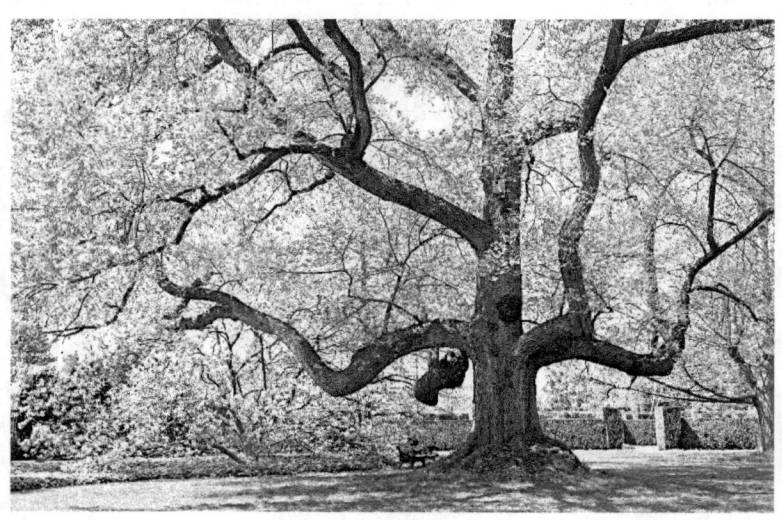

Acknowledgments

When I was 41, I had open-heart surgery to replace a crusted aortic valve. It had been degenerating for years, I assume, from the rheumatic fever I suffered in the refugee camp in Austria as a baby shortly after World War II. In 1985, the damage caught up with me. I could not walk upstairs without huffing and puffing, nor walk a city block without vomiting. It looked like I would be dead within the year. I was only 41!

I want to thank Dr. Barwynski, a heart surgeon, at St. Boniface Hospital in Winnipeg, who gave me a St. Jude Valve, size 23, which has gifted me with an additional 37 years of life, during which time I got married and have written some 30 odd books.

Dr. Barwynski, squeezed me in on a Sunday for my heart surgery using Canada's Universal Healthcare System, which made it possible for me not to go into a debt which could have taken years to pay off. If only the rest of the world would take care of its citizens that way, then the world might be a better place.

In 2017, I had another heart surgery to repair an aortic aneurysm. I was 71 at that time. Recovery was more difficult, as I came out of the hospital with bed sores.

I'd been put in a chair after surgery and went into a coma. Apparently, the nurses were short-staffed and did not turn me. Our universal healthcare system has been deteriorating for years and has, indeed, failed, as more people have huge wait times to deal with. The system is becoming more and more private.

I can see more and more people using the services of MAiD. Cancer has not been cured yet, nor other incurable diseases like Multiple Sclerosis, and Parkinson's. Who knows what pain people are suffering, how excruciating and chronic it is?

Indeed, if there is a way out, who can blame them? If I were in that blind alley of never-ending pain, I would seriously consider MAiD. I remember going under in 2017, prepped for my second heart surgery. A slipped into unconsciousness, into oblivion, waking up hours later to the words, "the operation was a success." I did not remember anything after being put under when I lost consciousness.

Maybe, the IV or needle they give you with MAiD is similar to what I experienced during my heart operation, absence of awareness, painless, where you sort of fall asleep. It's tempting to end one's pain that way if you have a terminal illness. Who knows what you would do, dear reader, if you had to face a terminal illness which involved daily terrible pain? Others do not understand!

The song says, "Nobody knows the pain I am in; nobody knows my sorrow." Indeed, that is so. We each must face our own death someday.

This may, ironically, be the last book that I will write. That reminds me of lyrics from a song by the Canadian band, Edward Bear, one of my favourite groups from the 1970s:

> So, I'll write you one more song
> But it's the last time that I'll ever try
> It's the last song I'll ever write for you.
>   *1972.*

In those days, I was hanging out at Tim Horton's after university, drinking coffee and reading <u>War and Peace</u>.

Now, after so many decades, there are too many things wrong with me to have any expectation to live another decade, though it would be nice to keep my wife company and maybe squeeze in writing another book or two.

My arrhythmia, my artificial heart valve, and my chronic leukemia may have other ideas. I've had several incidences already where the ambulance has had to be called. One of these days, I will experience terrible dizziness, a pain shooting down my left arm, turning purple like Mayor Meinzinger did when I saw him die during a presentation in grade 8, and finally, a loss of consciousness and separation from the world. Of course, MAiD may intervene before a natural death like that takes place. Perhaps, I can be spared all that pain.

The worry I have is that the policy and parameters of MAiD are controlled and administered by people who are young and healthy for those people who are not. I am 77 years old now. I walk through my fatality before me. Oh well!

Either way, what do my books matter now, any success I've had? We come into this world with nothing and leave with nothing. I often think of the lines in a western novel I wrote some years ago, where the trail boss says a prayer over the body of a cowboy who drowned in the Red River herding cattle in a storm:

> We brought nothing into this world, and we can carry nothin' out,
> the Lord gave and the Lord has taken away,
> Blessed be the name of the Lord.
>   Amen

[The Tipperary Kid, by John Hartig, 2019, publ. Through Amazon and Kindle.]

*****

I started writing seriously in 2008. My brother-in-law, Ken Janzen, had just died that winter, and people thought that someone should write a book on his agonizing journey of lung cancer. After all, there was so much said on his Blog and so many sentiments expressed! It was a shame to just let all that writing on the Blog disappear because nobody saved it. Since no one took up the chore, I took it on, writing a Trilogy entitled, <u>Time in a Bottle</u>. I don't think anyone's read it.

It's been 15 years, and I've notched up some 30 books in that time, available on Amazon and Kindle. My books are not literary masterpieces, but some are nicely done.

Why do I write? I think it's the same impulse as Anne Frank, who perished in a concentration camp at the hands of the Nazis.

"When I write I can shake off all my cares. My sorrow disappears, my spirits are revived."
ANNE FRANK

The Final Exit

Part I
Blessed are those...I suppose,
who can make their final exit,
in ripe old age and painless peace.
Ideally, that is the way we all should go,
with ease and peace, a slow deep sleep.
But reality, sadly, is not so!
Medical Assistance in Dying
is a preferred choice and ever growing.
It's a cure for terminal illness and constant pain.
Long-suffering these days could be in vain.
Why put up with it!
What a wonderful service to humanity!
Convenience in modern society!
But is it a good thing?
MAiD is expanding its definition,
ever increasing its merciful mission,
to include the irremediably mentally ill.
Soon perhaps, also the poor and homeless too?
And those disabled in wheelchairs,
It's scary, what if they were you!
Quality of life, a flexible commodity,
If government has no money,
no funds for humane programs,
forcing people to suffer in silent strife.
The old and sick have no choice,
in waiting lines, they have no voice,
helpless people are seduced by the tempting call,
of MAiD which promises to end it all.
And so it is, and so it is!

Part II
Hamlet asked disturbing questions,
Him: to be or not to be,
Us: to MAiD or not to MAiD?
If we removed all the unhappy people,
from the human race,
would that not make a better place?
Give us a pain-free death for our nation.
Surely, it's a blessed temptation.
To sleep? To dream? Or to go
to a country that we cannot see?
It could be heaven.
it could be hell.
We do not know.
Hamlet's dagger could have ended his life,
but with too much thinking, he did not act,
He endured his anguish and his strife.
He held on to kill the king, that scheming lout!
MAiD could have helped Hamlet out!
Dylan Thomas was an unrealistic poet,
raging against death, the dying of the light,
do not go gently, he said, into that good night.
Easy to say, if you are only 33!
There were poems yet to write,
as far as the eye could see.
Sunny days lay before him,
full of vigor and of vim,
satisfaction from ornamented words,
words that his poetry could sing,
and the money it could bring.
Dylan Thomas, Promethean,
raging against gods and demons alike,

angry at his brief mortality,
covetous of what he could not have -
ever grasping at out-of-reach eternity.
He did not see what old age,
was really like!
Stooped, reduced and feeble,
no choice, no voice to rave.
How could old age then be brave?
Dylan Thomas did not see clearly,
through his naive poetry,
that a warrior's cry is futile
against the dying of the light!
That nothing can be done
against relentless time.
Even in our raging prime,
we all will sadly someday end,
not with a bang,
but with a whimper.
and so it is, and so it is!

Part III
Dylan Thomas died of pneumonia,
only 39, when he breathed his last,
drunk on what he achieved in his past,
drunk on ego and too much whiskey.
He heedless of bad habits, so risky.
A stupor sank him into deep, deep sleep,
lulling him into a dizzy dream,
where nothing was real, so it would seem,
his true reality was a hospital bed,
A sad poet's death, a sober dread!
Caught in a coma, and finally death.
He had no choice, and no voice.
and so it was, and so it was.

Poor Dylan Thomas! No raging,
no raving, no rebelling.
He bragged rashly in his youthful pride,
"I've had 18 straight whiskies...
I think that's a record!"
The poor man, bloated, aged and worn,
before his time,
his body abused whilst in his prime.
Six drinks or eighteen?
All a braggart's lie!
What does a boast matter?
when you die?
Thomas was muddled on a murky road,
of self-destruction,
and like Jim Morrison,
another clever wordsmith
somewhat younger at 27,
both dying with no power to fight,
against death's insurmountable might.
We are all mortal riders of the storm!
Staving off the dying light,
We are no longer brave rebels,
who will not conform.
If overcome by old age,
we lose the youthful will to rage.
And so it is, and so it is!

Part IV
Age will not grant more afternoon delights,
No more burning Father Time at both ends,
no more Hope nor Faith to make amends.
There will be no more time,
to waste in our youthful prime!
Such a waste, oh what a waste!

To live a life in hedonistic haste!
A poet's soul is a divine gift of grace,
freely given to pass on to the human race.
And yet, if there is no wisdom in how to live,
Then there is sadly nothing there,
to pass on, to give.
There could have been so much more,
had they seen what to live for,
to share their art
 and their humanity,
as an immortal legacy.
But wasted, it was not meant to be,
Sadly, it was not so, it was not so.

John Hartig July 7, 2023

*There is nothing original in this poem. It is an aggregate of thoughts from Hamlet's Soliloquy, from Johnny Nash's song, I can see clearly now, and from Dylan Thomas' poem, do not go gentle into that good night.

John's Journal
Pre-Op

- Sept. 2023 200 beats
- Oct. 2023, ICD implant
- April 8, 2024, total Eclipse
- April 19, 2024, ABLATION
- May 17, 3:00 p.m., 2024, ICD shock

Where do I begin? The last 9 months have been miserable. It is June 4, 2024. At this juncture in my journal, I have lost my Muse. I cannot write. My imagination left me and my urge to write has flat-lined. I'm hoping that my health will get stronger from week to week and that my urge will come back.

I was scheduled for ablation surgery on April 19, 2024, which was supposed to correct my irregular heartbeat. I faced fatigue every day. I took morning and afternoon naps. Needless to say, I slept a lot accumulating unproductive days. My entry here, at the end of this book on MAiD, was supposed to simply include a "pre-op" preamble and a "post-op" wrap-up.

Well, the ablation did not work, so its failure necessitated a 90 degree turn in my writing. I would have been content to slog along with waves of energy and then doldrums, as long as my urge to write interrupted intermittently. But in September 2023, my heart had a health crisis. It raced up to 200 beats per minute and then plummeted to 30 beats, close to stopping. We called the ambulance and the next 9 months, as I said, were miserable. Since West Lincoln Hospital in Grimsby does not have cardiologists, I was transferred to Hamilton General at about 3:00 a.m. in a most uncomfortable and bumpy ride. Dr. Healey implanted an ICD which is supposed to be "the Cadillac" of devices, being both a pacemaker and defibrillator combo. "It'll save your life," he said. When I asked about the defibrillator part of it, he said, "Don't worry. You'll know when it kicks in." I was hoping that now I was taken care of, so that I could get back to my writing. I had a novel germinating in my mind. I didn't quite feel ready to write the first sentence. In the meantime, the world was waiting for the total eclipse of the sun. I think there was a song about that somewhere.

We were in a good position here in the Niagara Region to see this phenomenon as the moon crossed the sun's path at about 3:15 p.m. on Monday, April 8, 2024. I did not purchase special glasses, not needing to see the thing "in person". TV would be fine!

Hotels and motels in Niagara Falls were charging a thousand dollars a night in a true capitalistic spirit. That's amusing because the weather forecast called for overcast skies.

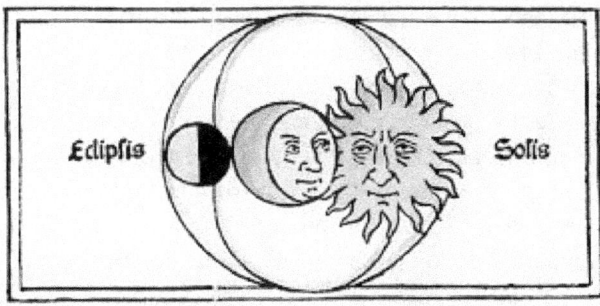

A TV network has seen fit to feature the disaster movie, "Meteor" that afternoon, maybe in keeping with cosmic events which affect the Earth. Another movie this weekend, on another channel, "Countdown Armageddon", also set the mood for huge solar/lunar events. Some religious extremists insisted that the eclipse symbolized God's displeasure with mankind. Bible thumpers proclaimed that the end of days were what we deserved. The CBC was tracking the sun's progress from Mexico and the U.S. right to Gander, Newfoundland.

My ablation was scheduled about two weeks after the total eclipse of the sun, specifically April 19, 2024. I had complete faith in what Dr. Healey was doing. My unruly heart presented him with a challenge. My artificial aortic valve was in the way of the filament which he'd guide to the parts of the heart which were causing the irregular rhythm. To get better angles on the situation, Dr. Healey decided to make entry on both sides of the groin. Since I was on the blood thinner, coumadin, the surgery required that my blood thinning be controlled, first to make it thicker and then after the ablation, to make it thin again. I had to inject Hepburn needles into my tummy twice a day. Ouch!

I incurred rheumatic fever in the refugee camp in Austria after WW II. The effect of rheumatic fever doesn't show until years later, in my case in 1987, at the age of 41 when I needed that aortic valve replaced...drastically! I never would have gotten around to writing some 30 odd books, had Canada's Universal Healthcare System not taken care of me then.

So, here I am so many years later, with the total eclipse of the sun crossing our path in Niagara with one more novel still unwritten, a mere idea in my mind.

I'm glad that Amazon gives me this chance to write and to publish for free. I enjoy designing my own book covers. I've had two books published through regular companies, The New Crusades, about an "honor-killing" through Tellwell, and its sequel, published in 2017 through Friesen Press, at a cost of several thousand dollars per shot, without marketing and publicity, which would again cost another couple of thousand dollars per book. With 30 books, you can imagine how much that would have cost me! So, I write for free without marketing.

Why do I do this? It is not for fame nor fortune. I have a ingrained need to write...and it's a way to keep busy in retirement.

Several other publishers have contacted me since Tellwell published my first murder mystery. They have a "hybrid" program now, where they pay half, and the author pays the other half for republishing and marketing a novel. I guess Amazon has put the squeeze on other publishing companies. I answered a phone call from America where a representative asked me if I still wanted to publish my book. I asked which one? He didn't know. Shoddy research on his part? I was not impressed and hung up.

I remember the days back in the 1950s when an author got paid a huge cheque up front if a book looked promising. Those days are gone.

Amazon deals with millions of authors world-wide. It seems like everybody's an author now-a-days. The New Crusades, publ. originally by Tellwell in 2015, is ranked 10,591,832 now on Amazon's reprint.   My best seller, The Final Exit, about the exponential growth of medical assistance in dying in Canada, is ranked 1,391,129. And my other best ranked, The Sasquatch Family, is ranked 4,030,760. I feel somewhat humbled by my rankings, and yet, I keep on cranking my books out because that, at my age of 78, gives me purpose and keeps me busy.

I had the notion once, that my topics were so unique that they'd be best sellers, but that is delusory! I wrote a Baroque murder mystery, for instance, on Who Killed Jean-Marie Leclair? Also, a history book which revisited the life of that Canadian Metis hero, Louis David Riel. Then, The Chosen, about the ownership of a Guarneri violin which traversed time through various owners from Vivaldi to the hands of a hippie in August 1969. But rather than be a victim to the changing tastes of my reading audience, I soldier on in my craft because I simply need to.

I saw a movie over the weekend prior to Monday's total eclipse of the sun. The title? "Writer Boy's Dream". I guess I'm sort of like that.

Young Malcolm Gross was not a practical boy. He was adamant that he had to be a writer. His destiny was to write. The problem, according to other people, was that the boy had no specific goal in mind about what to write, no genre, no category, no topics.

Caught in the foster system, he had no practical way of making his dream come true. I think, he was on the autistic spectrum. No, he had no specific genre in mind for writing, historical, crime, or fantasy. He simply wanted to write!

Reality smacked him in the face when a publisher said his company wanted to buy his book. The boy had talent! Malcolm sat in the publisher's office, so hopeful, and then, the man said the company wanted to buy his book, but without him!

Malcolm didn't understand. This was his book, his thoughts, his feelings wrenched out of his own life and gut! Yet, the publisher wanted to publish Malcolm's dream with another author's name on it because that would be a better marketing plan. Malcolm almost committed suicide. Later, his book, <u>Dream</u>, reached number one on Amazon, with his own name on it because he refused to give up his dream!

I intended to insert my unwritten book about the Milan prison in between my ablation pre-op experience and my post-op experience. But the whole thing rearranged itself when the ablation went awry. The idea for my unwritten book may be a golden one yet, if my Muse comes back to me. I got the idea from Mark Wigmore who hosts The Oasis program on 96.3 Classical FM radio. He recounted how prisoners in Milan made musical instruments out of derelicts which they used to cross the Mediterranean Sea to seek a better life in Italy. They were, in a sense, a new type of boat people. Being a refugee myself after WW II from Austria, I imagined myself as one of these boat people who was arrested after fleeing from the Middle East. Would such a story interest a reading audience who already listen to enough stories about the violence in Gaza and Ukraine?

This time, I said to myself, I needed to take more time to write such a story. Usually, I crank out a book every 6 months.

Of course, my intention to write this book may come to nothing, if I do not live through my upcoming ablation. As I said, I am scheduled for heart surgery in two weeks, April 19th, 2024. Let's hope that it is successful. If so, then my book will become a reality, and if not, then at least I've got 30 books already to my credit as a legacy.

I like the message in that movie about Malcolm. This message is highlighted in the lyrics of a song at the end:

"Yeah, your mind is a space that creates your horizons. Why would you look outside yourself when you have all of the world inside!"

Songwriters: Nathaniel Donnis / Kolby Knickerbocker

Ablation

This is written 7 days, one week, before my ablation. The procedure is scheduled for next Friday April 19th, 2024. I'm anxious about it. A younger man who had the same procedure the week before said that his surgery went smoothly. He'd only wished he'd worn sunglasses because of the bright lights in the operating room.

My case is more complicated. Nobody contacted us about whether I needed to do "bridging" for this surgery because I'm on a blood thinner. I need to transfer from coumadin to Hepburn, and after the surgery, back again to coumadin, all due to the fact that I have an artificial aortic heart valve. My wife had to phone the anesthesiologist and the surgeon's office twice to pursue the matter of whether I had to do bridging. Nothing can be taken for granted!

We've had this happen before with my hernia operation on the left side of my groin. The surgeon blithely went ahead with the surgery, stapled me up and sent me home. Within the week, my cut ballooned up and finally burst open at a clinic where I asked, "what's going on?" "Oh, you'd better clean up the mess and drive over to the specialist's office who did the surgery." When I got to the office, she looked at the open wound and asked, "What do you want me to do about it?" I said, "You're the doctor. I'm on coumadin. How do I stop the bleeding?" "Go to the drugstore across the street, buy Kotex napkins, wear them in your underwear until the wound heals." I don't know if she charged OHIP for this unscheduled visit. It took 4 months for my wound to close up. Nice scar! So, this time our persistence paid off because "bridging" was indeed necessary for this ablation.

If I lived through this operation, then there is a novel about the Milan prison within the intervening pages of this book. I didn't want to start it, not wanting to start something that I might not finish. I'm thinking this might also be my last book, having earned a paltry $700 over the past decade on about 30 other books I've churned out for Amazon. I've seen some of my books on Barnes and Noble and I suppose they are the ones collecting any profit from my books. At least, I'm publishing for free, and I guess that's just the price you have to pay.

I'm also thinking this might be my last book since I turned 78 years old two months ago. Most of my high school comrades have already passed away. Who knows when the bell will toll for me? I'm worried about dementia or Alzheimer's so that I won't be able to keep my thoughts straight to give a logical flow to this book of mine. Besides the topic of this book, Alzheimers' ironically can be a prison as well, because it is the dying of the light, the lack of energy falling away for research and mental activity to put words together. My imagination will be stretched thin to imagine characters in my novel about the Milan prison. Nothing is fair.

I am currently watching a movie starring Nicolas Cage, *Dying of the Light*, where he has onset dementia, and he is forced out of the secret service agency for blowing up at his boss who ignores clues that a terrorist has resurfaced after an absence of 22 years. If anything, the movie underscores the fact that ordinary people are victims to a bureaucratic machine working relentlessly above us of political agendas and ambitions of petty people who do not want to relinquish the reins of power. Nicolas Cage pursues an Arab terrorist despite the onset of his dementia: "Benir, you think you can hide? Nobody can hide from the Reaper!"

While I'm wrestling with imagining a world for the characters and events in my novel on the Milan prisoners, I hear that the Persians [Iran] in real-life news have launched missiles against Israel this week. Not the first time that has happened, this conflict. It happened in the Old Testament in the Book of Esther with Xerxes, the King of Persia, who held Hebrews in captivity. Iranians are indeed modern Persians. So, here we go again!

If this were my last week of life, I don't think I'd change anything. I have no bucket list, nor the health to pursue it. I'd still watch my YouTube movies. I'd still watch The View and get the latest gossip on Trump. It's always interesting to hear what Whoopi and the other ladies have to say about the crazy things happening in the world. What are the Americans going to do after Iran launched 300 missiles aimed at Israel. If I make it through my ablation surgery on Friday, it would be another lease on life for me. Maybe I'd try harder on my next novel to create a better product. I know I've also got another poem or two up my sleeve!

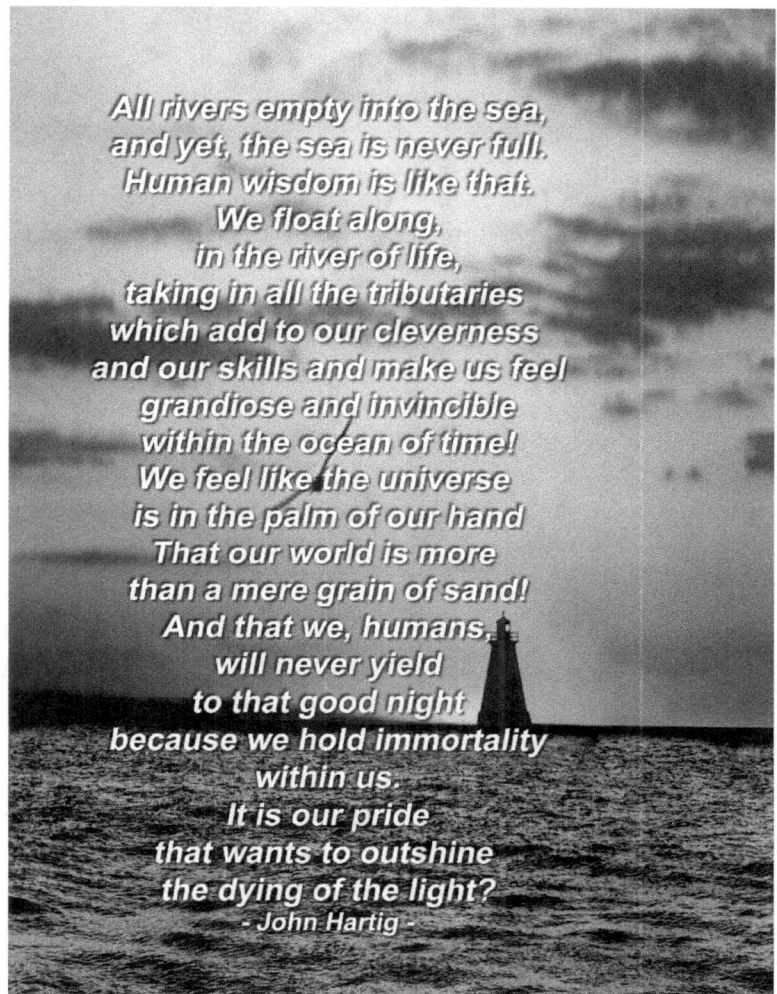

All rivers empty into the sea,
and yet, the sea is never full.
Human wisdom is like that.
We float along,
in the river of life,
taking in all the tributaries
which add to our cleverness
and our skills and make us feel
grandiose and invincible
within the ocean of time!
We feel like the universe
is in the palm of our hand
That our world is more
than a mere grain of sand!
And that we, humans,
will never yield
to that good night
because we hold immortality
within us.
It is our pride
that wants to outshine
the dying of the light?
- John Hartig -

I can't remember the last time I had a dream...until this week. There are some people who insist they have no regrets in life. Well, I take that with a grain of salt. I dreamt that an old girlfriend came into the office for a passport renewal. She wore the old school jacket, light blue with the school emblem on it. I was standing in line, face averted. I spotted her; she did not spot me. When she turned to look at some brochures on the wall, I snuck out and scurried away like a scared rabbit. I suppose I was not the one to leave a relationship without hard feelings. Maybe she was a better person than me. Strange how that goes. Who knows what my life might have been had I taken another road? Yet, I took the road I did and met my wife years later and for that, I am grateful.

It's ground 0. This is the evening before my surgery. The specialist says that the surgery will only improve my life 25%, which is better than nothing. I'll take it if I have more energy during the day. Right now, I feel dragged out and I need cat naps during the day, both at mid-morning and mid-afternoon. Not good! Especially, if you want to produce a novel! There are so many things yet to do in life and so much to read about and learn. In the face of death, people still want to cling on to their consciousness and to connected to the world. If you read this, it means I filled in the middle with an actual book. I hope it's been a worthwhile product.

John's Journal
Post-Op

- Sept. 2023 200 beats
- Oct. 2023, ICD implant
- April 8, 2024, total Eclipse
- April 19, 2024, ABLATION
- May 17, 3:00 p.m., 2024, ICD shock

The Morning After:

I'm home. It was a 3-hour surgery. Dr. Healey went in through the groin and threaded the filament up to the heart. Actually, he had to do both sides of the groin because my artificial aortic heart-valve was in the way. The EKG before the procedure showed A-Fib, a couple of PVCs, peaks, valleys and craters, as my wife calls them on the read-out, but when Dr. Healey was in there, they were not evident, so he could not see what to zap with the laser. It's like when you have a rattle in your car engine, you take it into the mechanic and the engine noise disappears! Sigh!

Dr. Healey did not burn or ablate anything so as not to damage the heart further. I've already had two open-heart surgeries, one for the valve when I was 41 and then more recently, for an aortic aneurysm repair when I was 71. Dr. Healey figures since the weather is getting warmer, my body will get more stamina with a little walking outdoors. So, there you go, I made it through!! If I have future incidences, this alation procedure may be done again! Sigh!!

This non-ablation procedure left me with a few problems which required another two and a half weeks stay at the Hamilton General Hospital. When I woke up, I my left leg was black and blue from my butt down to my ankle. The right leg had no trouble healing within the usual two-day period.

However, the left leg presented the problem. I had an internal bleed. My femoral artery had a six-inch tear in it after the procedure. I could have died. Two surgeons had to apply manual pressure on the left side of my groin for half an hour to get the bleed to stop. I got close to losing my life in a surgery which was supposed to be simple. Well, for other people! I had to get used to the hospital food at the Hamilton General over the next two and a half weeks.

My ICD:

I was glad to be back home but May 17th, 2024 held another surprise for me. I was dropping off to sleep at 3:00 p.m., a nice afternoon nap when I got the most excruciating shock I'd ever experienced in my chest. "Marjorie," I yelled. "Heart-attack!"

I'd been told what the defibrillator part of my new device would feel like, if it went off. Yes, like a horse kicking you in the chest. We are used to calling the ambulance now if something happens; otherwise, we wait for hours in the Emergency Ward of the hospital. The extra charge of $45 for ambulance service is worth the faster attention. We went to the St. Catharines General this time. I had to get used to the hospital food there over the next two and a half weeks. It was comforting to know that the cardiologist at St. Catharines conferred with Dr. Healey at the Hamilton General. I had to go through the whole routine of balancing my coumadin off with Hepburn shots in my stomach, so that my blood thinning would settle down at 2.5.

I had no complaints about the hospital food. I was fed and kept alive! It was the nights which were difficult. Ambient noise all around and my roommate's sojourns to the washroom, leaving the light on, which kept me awake. The hours dragged by from pain med to pain med when I could ask for another pill to dull my senses.

I was glad when my INR hit 2.5 and the doctor gave the okay to go home. Home: for my own sitting room, my own meals, my own bathroom, my own TV and my own bed. There's no place like home!

I thought of writing something, but it feels like a heavy leaden weight is holding me back. It's going to be slow slogging to stoke the embers for my writing fire.

Flashbacks

They say that your life flashes before you when you die. I don't know what my very last thoughts will be, but these last few months have been a review of salient moments in my life, moments I might have changed and moments for which I have regret.

I was married previously. I'd always carried an invisible inferiority sign on my back hailing back to my elementary school days as a refugee. I'd been put back to grade 1 as an 8-year-old to learn English and the system simply kept me there. My average of 90% did not make a difference to my life at that stage. Jim Moyer edged me out at 91%. Both of us ended up in grade 9A at St. Jerome's High, an all-boys Catholic school. The school was streamed according to intelligence and achievement. Jim scored high in the sciences throughout high school; I got 55% in grade 12 Math. He, along with the other clever kids in my class became engineers, doctors, lawyers and accountants. I took the double honours English and History program. I never valued my degree and wasted a lot of time in the coffee shop. Jim, by the way, died of cancer at the age of 69. He left some landmark buildings behind in his architectural career. Jim got married in 1972 when I still did not know what to do with my life. When he died in 2018, one can only guess how he coped with dying. I wondered if he might have chosen to use MAiD because it was available then but then Catholics thought suicide was a sin.

When I got married, I had a job as a reporter for the Chilliwack Progress. I was making half her salary. When my first wife asked if it would be alright for her coworker at the town's planning commission to move into the rooms downstairs in the old farmhouse where we were renting, I should have seen alarm bells go off. They had an affair. I should never have gotten married, not at that time, until I found a more secure career path.

I moved to Grande Prairie where I landed a job as the editor of Grande Prairie This Week. I was single again but felt stuck in a low-paying job because publishers paid their staff peanuts in those days. I worked 60 hours a week and held bitterness in my heart, not wanting to get into any relationship again.

I am grateful to my brother for moving in with me to prevent me from doing anything foolish. And also, the psychologist, Claire Weeks, who wrote Hope and Help for Your Nerves, which gave me insights into depression which clouded my outlook in those dark days.

I__ entered my life when I was recovering and trying to heal my shattered life. She said, "Please, don't hurt me." I hugged her and didn't say a thing. Months went by. I became uneasy about "commitment". I tore that relationship apart. My bitterness over my failed marriage boiled in the hidden recesses of my mind. Quitting my editor's job at the newspaper and entering a first-year apprenticeship program as an electrician did not solve anything either. I had a pinched herniated disc which made that job impossible. I broke it off with I__. I'm sorry I hurt you.

E___ entered my life next. I floated along in that relationship without committing. She gave me an ultimatum; I ignored it. She did what was best for herself, first leaving the school in which we both taught; then, registering herself in a PhD program at the University of Calgary to eventually become a professor. E___ could do the Rubik's Cube in 3 minutes to the astonishment of all her students. I felt deep-down insignificant. I knew she would go on to bigger and better things. Our destinies headed in different directions. She was too clever for me; I felt insecure.

I had a nervous breakdown. With meds and counseling, I got onto the road to recovery. I sold the house and registered at the Winnipeg Bible College to search for God. When I met my current wife, I'd already gone through a regimen of meds and intense counseling.

I prayed and felt that she was someone God had meant for me. Both of us saw Paris in the springtime during my university stint in France in 1989. We also rented a car and drove through Germany and Austria. It was a great summer before we were hired at Niagara Christian College.

I am grateful to the Mennonite church in Grande Prairie and in Winnipeg, people who spent time with me during my recovery during my nervous breakdown, encouraging me to seek God and not be pulled back into my old battle with the Devil. Marjorie agreed to take care of collecting the rent for my house. Selling it gave me the funds for my studies at the Canadian Mennonite Bible College in Winnipeg. I switched to French by taking on French courses through the University of Winnipeg. It had an exchange program with the Universite de Perpignan in southern France. What a great idea to get my BA in French. Although not official, my wife was counted as the 20th student in this program so that we had the go ahead. Marjorie had to sign all kinds of papers not to work in France and not to take anybody's job.

Niagara Christian College only lasted two years since the enrolment there dropped off. I agreed to teach elementary school in Foleyet, a little village an hour and a half outside of Timmins. Just when I accepted that job, a phone call came in to teach overseas in a private American school in Hungary. I felt honor bound, however, to follow through on the Foleyet job which was a big mistake. We should have gone to Budapest. The principal at Foleyet was domineering and mercurial about changing my assignments. After a stressful two years, my wife and I moved back to Fort Erie. I took on substitute teaching jobs around Niagara. My wife got hired full time for the Niagara School District while I was sporadically called to fill in as substitute teacher.

It was Marjorie's full time employment which gave me the chance to enroll at Mohawk College at night school. I got a certificate in web design. I also took on a couple of part-time gigs as a wedding photographer. Later, I restricted my photography to scenery, sunsets and flowers. I published several very nice photobooks on <u>The Niagara Peninsula: Land of Wineries and Orchards</u>.

I found it ironic to design web sites during my retirement after I said I hated computers. That is how I write my novels now and design them, including the book covers, amassing over 30 photobooks and novels of various genres, all available on Amazon. I'm glad I lived this long to do that.

My classmates were so fortunate to be born in Canada. After WW II in the refugee camp in Austria, I inherited health problems. I survived rheumatic fever, which of course, showed up later in Canada as a damaged aortic valve which needed replacing. I also survived two years in a sanatorium for tuberculosis in Austria. Canada was a saving grace. If only the rest of the world could even out the wealth and health in all countries. The planet has so much potential which we all could enjoy if only religion and nationalism did not get in the way.

Anyway, I pray that my irregular heartbeat does not give me a stroke and that my brain remains clear when I get the urge to pursue my passion for writing. It's amazing how your brain and body can replace things in your life when things are taken away from you. Thank God for computers, after all!

I'm more open to medical assistance in dying than Jim might have been. My concept of God certainly does not fall in line with what the Church preaches. I don't think of him as a benevolent father with a white beard sitting on a cloud and I don't think of him as an ethereal energy source. He is a concept though, which will help me die and bear up to the trials in life. He is the most-hoped-for best in humanity when we swear to something. He is an idea of the best in whatever we are.

I imagine my heart will be the death of me. A heart attack or a stroke. A dizzy spell, fainting, falling, passing out and then, Blackness! I've tried to make friends with Jesus several times during the night when I felt despair or loneliness. Even if Jesus were not the third person of the Trinity, I'd rather have him as a friend than the false prophets in finance or politics. I pray that when I die, Jesus is on the other side, to say, welcome, let's talk!

*****

To be or not to be. That is the question. If I suffered from an incurable illness and one that was painful throughout its stages to the end, I would consider medical assistance in dying. Provided that it was painless, like going to sleep. However, recent research has put doubts on that assertion. A recent article in LifeSiteNews, "Paralyzed then drowned", explained by Kelsi Sheren to Jordan Peterson that drugs are used to paralyze euthanasia patients and then drown them in their own fluids. It's equivalent to waterboarding. Sheren compared the procedure to the Nazis, once the patient is "completely paralyzed, then this drug is administered as one of the four and they start drowning to death." [LifeSiteNews: Wed 29, 2024]

If that is the case, then of course I would reject MAiD because who wants to drown to death? I am not confident that the medical system has done its complete research to make me feel comfortable that a patient indeed experiences a "painless compassionate death."

Both my wife and I have finally been accepted at the Regional Pain Clinic, that is after a three-year waiting list. When I had my appointment, I was cheerfully met by my pain doctor. I mentioned all my chronic aches and pains, my incurable knees and shoulders. When I mentioned that I had written a book on medical assistance in dying, the doctor perked up and wanted to show me that MAiD was available right there in that facility. I felt like I faced a promotional commercial. My wife and I did not like that. I declined the little tour.

With the few visits we've had to the pain clinic so far, we find that there is no miracle cure there! We were hoping, at least, for pain management but alas, no such management! The system, I feel is broken! But it's willing to put you in line to put you away, to help you die with needles. Certainly, more economical than long-term care! Reminds me of an old Charlton Heston movie I saw a long time ago, *Soylent Green*. We have Paradise in our hands, but we are sadly mismanaging.

Acknowledgements

When I was 41, I had open-heart surgery to replace a crusted aortic valve. It had been degenerating for years, I assume from the rheumatic fever I suffered in the refugee camp in Austria as a baby shortly after World War II. In 1985, the damage caught up with me. I could not walk upstairs without huffing and puffing, nor walk a city block without vomiting. It looked like I would be dead within the year. I was taking religious courses at CMBC at the time in Winnipeg in search of God.

I want to thank Dr. Barwynski, a heart surgeon, at St. Boniface Hospital in Winnipeg, who gave me a St. Jude Valve, size 23, which has gifted me with an additional 37 years of life, during which time I got married and have written some 30 odd books.

Dr. Barwynski, squeezed me in on a Sunday for my heart surgery using Canada's Universal Healthcare System, which made it possible for me not to go into a debt which could have taken me years to pay off. If only the rest of the world would take care of its citizens that way, then the world might be a better place.

I also want to thank Michael Kositsky for proof-reading the first ever novel I wrote in 2014, *The New Crusades*, and making excellent editorial suggestions for it.

My teachers at St. Jerome's High in Kitchener encouraged me in my academic pursuits and gave me a good classical education in the 1960s.

First of all, my English teacher, Mr. William Klos, who ignited a love of literature in me and who read poetry and excerpts with feeling. Also, Mr. Ronald Haston, who made history come alive, especially with his narrations and spirited introductions to every history class.

Thanks also to my wife. By the way, she likes to remain anonymous and prefers me not to name her. She lets me sneak off at midnight, close the bedroom door, and fire up the computer with a cup of tea by my side so I can write. Insomnia has its good points.

I liked the old way of having the publisher bear the expenses with a nice royalty check for the creator of the work. That was a good incentive for a writer.

Publication Contributions:
by John Hartig

1. Poem by John Hartig p. 43, "I Walked to Kenny's Grave Today", <u>Solitude: A Collection of New Canadian Poetry</u>, publ. 2009, Polar Expressions Publishing, Maple Ridge, BC.

2. Poem by John Hartig, "Songs of Innocence and Experience", <u>The Journey: A Collection of New Canadian Poetry</u>, publ. 20010, Polar Expressions Publishing, Maple Ridge, BC.

3. Short story by John Hartig, "Coffee Break", <u>Formation: New Canadian Short Stories</u>, publ. 2010, Polar Expressions Publishing, Maple Ridge, BC.

4. Short story by John Hartig, "Courage Getting Old", <u>From Across the River</u>, publ. 2011, Poetry Institute of Canada, Victoria B.C.

5. Center Page Photo Spread: <u>Our Canada – A Country for All Seasons</u>, "Spring Blossoms in Niagara-on-the-Lake," publ. 2012

6. Photo Design Ad Published: ARABELLA, Magazine Publication of Canadian Art, Architecture and Design, "Spring Awakenings 2012 Edition", Full page photo ad for *Granny's Boot Antiques* in Vineland, "Unique Folk-Art, Vibrant and Alive!" John Hartig Photos.

My Books

Fiction

The New Crusades, John Hartig, second ed. 2021, first publ. 2015, by Tellwell, under my penname, Waldemar Guenter, avail. through Amazon and Ingram

The New Crusades: The Sequel, John Hartig, second ed. 2021, first publ. by Friesen Press, 2016, under my pennames of Waldemar Guenter and Alexander Kucharski, avail. through Amazon and Ingram

Duplicity, publ. Amazon, 2018, John Hartig. avail. through Amazon and Ingram

Who Killed Jean-Marie Leclair? A Baroque Murder Mystery, publ. Amazon, 2019, John Hartig. avail. through Amazon and Ingram

Love and Faith Trilogy, Books I, II, III, publ. Amazon, 2019, John Hartig. avail. through Amazon and Ingram

The Polish Cowboy, publ. Amazon, 2019, John Hartig. avail. through Amazon and Ingram

The Tipperary Kid, publ. Amazon, 2019, John Hartig. avail. through Amazon and Ingram

John's Shorts: Little Stories with Big Ideas, publ. Amazon, 2022, John Hartig. avail. through Amazon and Ingram

John's Hidden Gems: Short Story Collection, publ. Amazon, 2022, John Hartig. avail. through Amazon and Ingram

Things Have Gotta Get Better Than This, publ. Amazon, 2022, John Hartig. avail. through Amazon and Ingram

The Chosen: A Violin Story, publ. Amazon, 2022, John Hartig. avail. through Amazon and Ingram

Adam's Journey, publ. Amazon, 2022, John Hartig. avail. through Amazon and Ingram.

Johann Joachim Quantz, Gift of the Flute, publ. 2022, John Hartig, avail. through Amazon and Ingram.

The Sasquatch, publ. 2023, John Hartig, avail. through Amazon and Ingram.

Non-Fiction

Time in a Bottle Trilogy, Books I, II, III, publ. Amazon, 2019, John Hartig. avail. through Amazon.

You Love Our Milk and Honey, Book I, II, publ. Amazon, 2020, John Hartig. avail. through Amazon.

The Second Wave: Living Through Trump and Covid, publ. Amazon, 2021, John Hartig. avail. through Amazon.

77 Looking Back: My Sort of Diary 2022-2023, publ. Amazon, 2023, John Hartig, avail. through Amazon.

The Final Exit: Medical Assistance in Dying, MAiD in Canada, publ. Amazon, 2023, John Hartig, avail. through Amazon.

Other

Can You Imagine? A children's picture book with poetry, publ. Amazon, 2019, John Hartig. avail. through Amazon and Ingram

Poetry Like Raindrops, publ. Amazon, 2019, John Hartig. avail. through Amazon and Ingram

Battle of the Violins, publ. Amazon, 2019, John Hartig. avail. through Amazon and Ingram

John's Photobook Series, Ball's Falls to Niagara Falls, publ. Amazon, 2021, John Hartig Photos. avail. through Amazon and Ingram

Louis Riel and Me, publ. Amazon, 2021, John Hartig, a historical fiction. avail. through Amazon and Ingram

Give Us Hopes and Dreams, publ. Amazon, 2021, John Hartig. avail. through Amazon and Ingram

Where Do Good Atheists Go? publ. Amazon, 2021, John Hartig. avail. through Amazon and Ingram

We Are Not Alone: Civilizations in Outer Space publ. Amazon, 2022, John Hartig. avail. through Amazon and Ingram.

The Cosmos: Origins and Aliens, publ. Amazon, 2022, John Hartig. avail. through Amazon and Ingram.

Johann Joachim Quantz, publ. Amazon, 2022, John Hartig, avail. through Amazon.

Two Baroque Prodigies, "Quantz flute tutor for Frederick the Great, Leclair, violinist murdered in 1764", publ. Amazon, 2022, John Hartig, avail. through Amazon.

*****

John's Photobook Series

I am proud, not only to have published numerous novels and short stories, but to have also published a whole series of Photobooks, showing off choice scenery, flowers and sunsets.

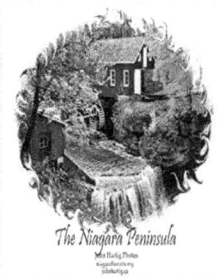

Photobooks are 8.5x8.5"

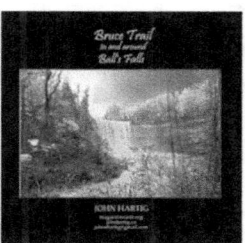

The Bruce Trail

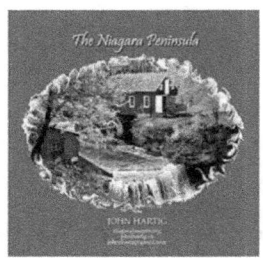

The Niagara Peninsula

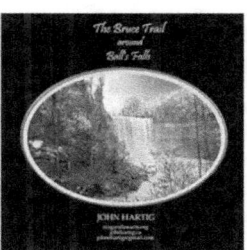

Ball's Falls

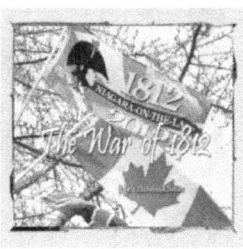

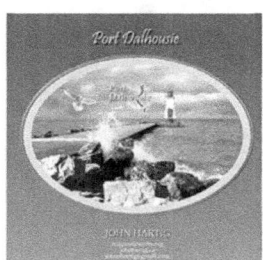

Port Dalhousie

The War of 1812

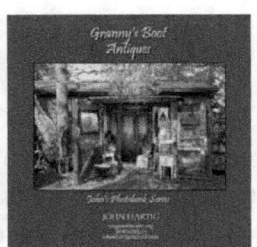

Granny's Boot Antiques

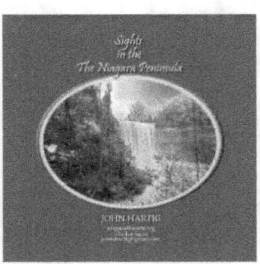

Sights in the
Niagara Peninsula

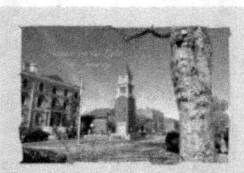

Niagara-on-the-Lake

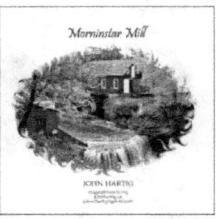

Morningstar Mill

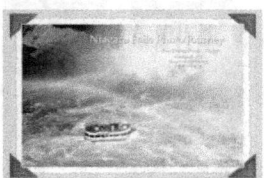

Niagara Falls

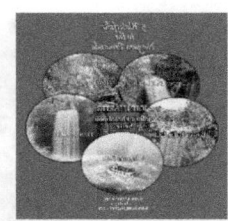

5 Waterfalls in Niagara

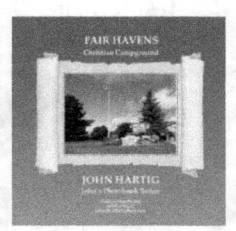

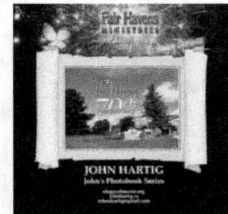

Fair Havens

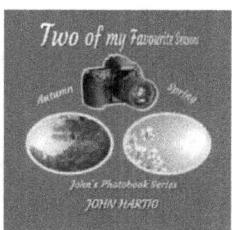

Two of my Favourite Seasons

70th Anniversary

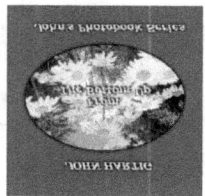

From The Bottom Up

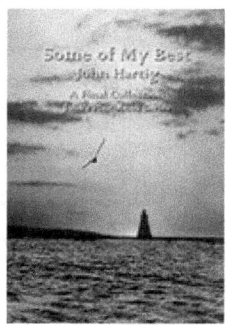

Some of My Best

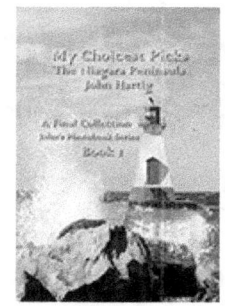

My Choicest Picks 1

*****

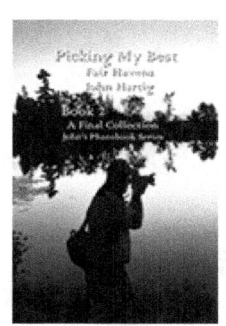

My Choicest Picks 2

*****

- ➤ John Hartig Novels through Amazon and Ingram, google title and John Hartig
- ➤ John's Photobook Series ordered directly from Amazon and Ingram.
- ➤ Prints, any size enlargements, e-mail John directly to place an order. Pickup at the house, otherwise + shipping cost

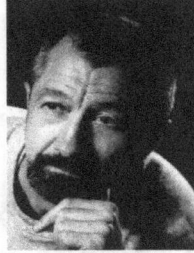

John Hartig

John lives in Vineland, Ontario. Photobooks and prints are available for home or office.

CONTACT
johnehartig@gmail.com
johnhartig.ca
Or just Google
John Hartig Novels or
Photography

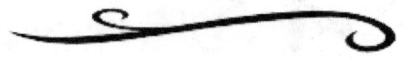

www.ingramcontent.com/pod-product-compliance
Lightning Source LLC
Chambersburg PA
CBHW072141290526
45794CB00004B/1385